Dear Friend,

Thank you for being part of Pressure Point Therapy. This is a wonderful technique that you will find easy to learn and apply. You'll get fantastic results with your friends, your family and with yourself.

As Pressure Point Therapy is a learning experience, I invite you to join me at **pressurepointtherapy.com**

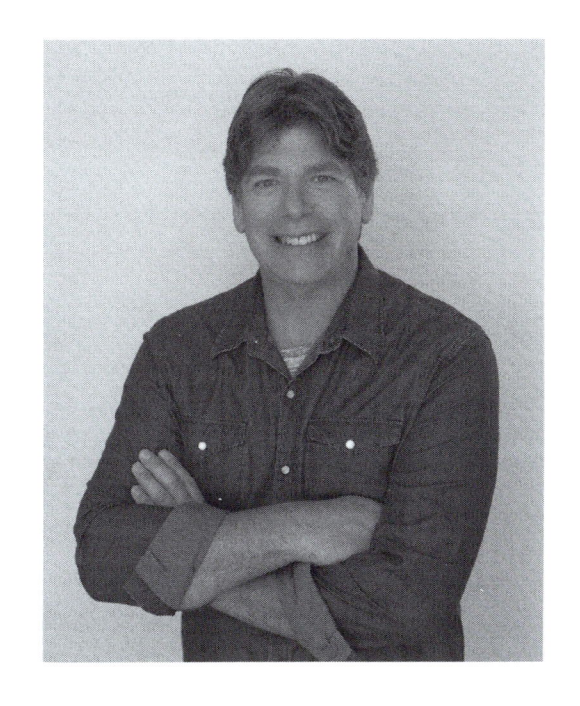

Here you will find the latest information, webinars and special offers. In fact, by signing up for my free newsletter you will receive 3 of my special reports on pain, sleep and nutrition--all at no charge. Simply follow the prompts to register on the web site.

You can always be connected with me at my Facebook page

facebook.com/drpinkus

The tools are in this book. Learn them. Apply the technique. Get great results!

In Health,
Dr. Michael Pinkus

PRESSURE POINT THERAPY

The complete do-it-yourself treatment manual

DR. MICHAEL PINKUS

Alternative Health Press

Alternative Health Press

Copyright © 2019, Dr. Michael Pinkus

All rights reserved. No part of this book may be reproduced in any form, or by any means, without permission in writing from the author.

PRESSURE POINT THERAPY® is a Registered Trademark

DR. MICHAEL PINKUS® is a Registered Trademark

Library of Congress Control Number: 2012942761

ISBN 978-0-9640393-2-2

Printed in the USA

www.pressurepointtherapy.com

www.facebook.com/drpinkus.com

www.alternativehealthpress.com

The information in this book is not meant to substitute for qualified medical care. If you are in need of medical attention, seek the advice of your chiropractor or medical doctor. The FDA has not evaluated the data in this book for accuracy.

Design and Layout: David Rilke www.davidrilke.com

Model renders courtesy of BodyParts3D, © The Database Center for Life Science licensed under CC Attribution-Share Alike 2.1 Japan

Editor: Jordin J. Pinkus

DEDICATION

To my beautiful wife and son. Your love, caring and support of me make this book and project possible. There will be many others thanking you as well.

TABLE OF CONTENTS

Part I: The Basics of Wellness — 1

Preface — 3

Chapter 1: Pressure — 6

Chapter 2: Rating Your Health—The Wellness Scale — 9

Chapter 3: Applying Pressure Point Therapy — 17

Chapter 4: How to Find Pressure Points — 20

Chapter 5: Pressure Points—How to Treat — 22

Chapter 6: Body Landmarks — 26

Chapter 7: The ABC's of Applying Pressure Point Therapy — 28

Chapter 8: Frequency of Treatment — 31

Chapter 9: Precautions — 32

Chapter 10: Do-It-Yourself Pressure Point Massagers and Devices — 34

Chapter 11: Nutrition — 37

Chapter 12: Taking Care of Your Body — 39

Part II: The Pressure Point Treatment Charts — 41

The Pressure Point Therapy Treatment Charts — 43

General Pressure Points For Greater Energy And Vitality — 44

Low-Back, Sciatic and Hip Pain Pressure Points — 46

Low Energy Pressure Points	48
Neck Pain Pressure Points	50
Upper- or Mid-Back Pain, Pain-Between-The-Shoulders Pressure Points	52
Pressure Points for Lung Problems	54
Pressure Points for Hand, Wrist and Elbow Pain	56
Pressure Points for Sinuses, Allergies, Head Colds and Congestion	58
Headache and Jaw Pain (TMJ) Pressure Points	60
Pressure Points for Hormonal Conditions (PMS, etc.)	62
Pressure Points for Digestive Problems	64
Pressure Points for Shoulder Pain	66
Knee Pain Pressure Points	68
Pressure Points for Cold and Flu Symptoms	70

About the Author   **73**

PART I: THE BASICS OF WELLNESS

PREFACE

We live in a country that is statistically one of the unhealthiest places to live on this planet.

One hundred years ago, the United States of America was the crown jewel of health. Today we are amongst the worst. Yet, we spend more on "health care" than any other country. One could look at these statistics and conclude that something is wrong.

There *is* something wrong: the American public (and inhabitants of other countries in similarly bad shape) have not received the entire story of how to take care of themselves and their families. There is simply missing data. My intention in writing this book is to fill this gap with *applicable* information regarding health care.

I have been studying and practicing Alternative Health Care for the past thirty years. Alternative Health Care is defined as the science and application of those techniques to treat the human body which do not include the use of drugs and/or surgery.

Years ago, it was unpopular to be involved with Alternative or Natural Health Care. In fact, I have been personally blasted by others for my studies and interest in this topic, being told "Alternative Health Care doesn't work," or "Why don't you become a real doctor." (I am a Doctor of Chiropractic.)

Today it is an entirely different story. People by the droves are actively seeking Alternative Health methods.

According to the National Institute of Health (NIH), four in ten people partake in natural health techniques in this country. Even the Pentagon is researching alternatives to traditional medicine—exploring techniques for post-traumatic stress disorder and several other conditions affecting our soldiers.

Of the dozens of Alternative Health Care techniques I have explored, many of these "alternatives" hold the key to the *actual reason* a person is sick or not doing well. There is no monopoly on health, even though there is an apparency that traditional medicine is the only choice.

As an example, I was doing a photo shoot the other day and the photographer told me he had "bursitis in the hip" for about six months. And even after medications and months of physical therapy, he was still in pain.

It didn't make sense to me that "bursitis" would persist that long, especially after this extensive treatment. So I decided to check out if he had Pressure Points in the area. I had him lie down on the floor of the photo studio (once you learn Pressure Point Therapy you can do it anywhere). I checked out the Pressure Points shown in the chart "Low-Back, Sciatic and Hip Pain Pressure Points" (this chart and several others are located in Part II of this book). There were at least six "blown" (active) Pressure Points. I treated the photographer using the techniques outlined in this book. The treatment took maybe four to five minutes. When I was done, he stood up and had no pain at all! He sent me a follow-up email and told me he was still pain-free! He couldn't believe it.

The point is "Alternative" Health is not *alternative* at all. It does not mean something "different" or something "out-there." Alternative Health, specifically Pressure Point Therapy, can often times be a primary or basic treatment system that gets to the root of many problems. I have had patients over the years who have had surgeries, numerous prescriptions, physical therapy, finally to be told, "You have to live with it." After all of that, a technique as simple as Pressure Point Therapy did the trick!

If I had not reset this photographer's circuit breakers (i.e. treated his Pressure Points) in his lower back and hip, he would have been hobbling along for the next thirty years. It wasn't simply a "good idea" to treat these points; he had a *mechanical problem* (the Pressure Points) shutting down the nerves in his low-back, hip and leg. Left untreated, his knee may have blown out, he could have developed a disc problem in his lower back or much more.

The same holds true for nutrition and other Alternative Health practices: a lack of just one nutrient in the body can affect so many systems that the person can go "head-over-green-tea" and develop all sorts of "medical conditions."

Then the obvious solution would be to replenish the nutrient and the problems would go away, right? Yes.

But in today's world, this person would go to a doctor complaining of X, Y and Z, have a series of tests done and most likely be put on several medications, all competing to destroy the liver and other organs while "suppressing" the symptoms. This person would end up even sicker or dead.

By the way, beware of doctors who give you a diagnosis that sounds like a prison sentence. These include the conditions that end in "-itis" (arthritis, bursitis, etc.) and those that end in "-algia" (neuralgia, fibromyalgia, etc.) The suffixes "-itis" and "-algia" mean "inflammation" and "pain" respectively.

Pressure Point Therapy was derived from techniques that date back over four thousand years. These include acupressure, acupuncture and shiatsu.

I practiced acupuncture for a time and found that people didn't like needles. Acupressure and shiatsu are great, but they require learning Oriental/Asian techniques, along with their philosophies and languages, which can be a challenge.

When I was studying these techniques, I started comparing the Asian acupuncture charts to the Western nerve charts of the body. I began to cross-reference which nerve pathways were involved with the ancient acupressure points. Where did the nerve travel to? What area of the body did it control or influence? Which organs were influenced by these points and how did this correspond to the nerve pathways in the body?

From these observations and many years of hands-on application, I derived this technique, which I coined "Pressure Point Therapy."

What's nice about Pressure Point Therapy is that anyone can learn it, apply it and get results. You don't have to have a medical background, be a doctor or have a PhD. In fact, some of the best "hands" I've experienced are from those who were complete medical laymen, with no training at all! You WILL learn this technique from this book and become GOOD at it, I promise.

There is another interesting phenomenon that I have observed from having taught this technique and having been on over one thousand radio and TV talk shows. That is, I see that almost everyone has a deep-rooted desire to *help others*. I can attest that there is no better feeling than helping another feel better almost immediately after applying Pressure Point Therapy. You will experience this too once you start applying this technique.

Another win that many experience is having and knowing the actual tools to help others. Being in control over an area, such as health care, gives one a true sense of Power!

Pressure Point Therapy is actually a lost art or ritual, especially in the Western world. It is my purpose, with this book and training materials, to bring it back in vogue.

Pressure Point Therapy is not difficult to learn or apply. You'll find it is somewhat innate or intuitive. It is not unlike observing an animal care for her pups. She doesn't have to "think about it." She just does it.

I have observed, in fact, that most people actually "treat" their own Pressure Points daily, without even knowing it. For example, rubbing one's forehead to relieve head-tension or reaching around and rubbing the top of the shoulder: one is treating his own Pressure Points! There are many other intuitive applications of this technique as well.

Is Pressure Point Therapy, therefore, a lost art? As we say in Minnesota, "You betch-ya!"

I believe that we human beings can do a lot with our hands to help others. You know the power of a hug, a pat on the back or a good, firm handshake. But with regards to Pressure Point Therapy, we have lost the know-how, the technology of application over the millennia. I'm not referring to esoteric practices of "healing with the hands" or "changing one's energy or aura" or any other so-called metaphysical techniques. What I am saying is that we can, with the instructions in this book, do a lot to help our fellow human beings.

I hope you're getting excited to continue reading this book and learning Pressure Point Therapy for yourself.

This manual was written and assembled with the purpose of you being able to easily read it and apply it. Use it. You will be amazed!

Dr. Michael Pinkus

CHAPTER 1: PRESSURE

We are all under pressure. Pressure is another word for stress. When a person thinks of stress, he thinks of the things which cause the stress: job, children, relationships, money, time, etc.

One can cope with stress to a degree. Some people do better than others. Every person has his own "stress threshold." If one stays within this threshold, the body functions normally. But when the pressures of the world go beyond this point, the stress infiltrates (gets into the body), and a person feels "stressed out." Most diseases in the body can be traced to stress or pressure, to one degree or another.

Pressure Point Therapy could have been called *Stress* Point Therapy. But it is important to differentiate between stress (which most people consider mental stress) and pressure, which is a physical thing. This pressure actually exists and it is wreaking havoc with your body.

Pressure Points

Your body stores "stress" in areas called Pressure Points. Pressure Points are small painful pockets of energy that are located around a nerve or along a nerve pathway in the body. Pressure Points will block the nerve energy from flowing through your body.

As you may know, your entire body is run by nerves. These nerves control all functions in your body. They run your heart, digestive system, muscles, immune system, senses of sight, taste, hearing, etc. If a nerve is blocked by a Pressure Point, the messages that flow through the nerve also become stopped or reduced.

For example, if you have a nerve that is responsible for your digestive tract and it is blocked by a Pressure Point, you may end up with indigestion, constipation or even diarrhea. Pressure Points blocking the nerves going into the head can result in headaches, neck pain or perhaps vision disturbances.

Pressure Points are located within and around the muscles in your body. Many of these nerves run directly through the muscles. This is especially true in your back. As you may know, your back contains the spinal column, which houses eighty percent of all the nerves in your body. Therefore, your back contains hundreds of Pressure Points.

How Pressure Points Form

When your body gets stressed out, your muscles tighten up. Many of you regularly feel this in your neck and shoulder areas. This stress can be either conscious or unconscious. When the muscles tighten up, they exert pressure on the nerves, which run through the muscle.

Nerves have an "Achilles heel." Where there is *any* pressure on a nerve whatsoever, the nerve goes into "red alert" and shuts down. "Pressure" here could be as extreme as getting hit by a bus or as simple as getting into an argument with your boss.

In either example, the nerve sends an "emergency" signal back to your brain, which, in turn, further tightens up the muscles. This results in a small area of extreme tightness, which we call a Pressure Point.

Because the nerves in the body are interconnected, a Pressure Point blocking a nerve in one area in the body can block the function of another part of the body.

For example, if a person has a Pressure Point in the upper back he may have back pain. The person can also develop difficulty in his lungs. Why? Because the nerve branches out into other areas.

If, in this example, the nerves are blocked to the lungs, what kind of problems do you think this person can have? That's right—lung congestion, bronchitis, or even pneumonia or asthma.

The basic idea then in Pressure Point Therapy is to find the area of Pressure Points and treat them to open up the nerve pathways again.

Road Map

Because of the anatomy of the body, it is easy to associate certain Pressure Points with different problems.

For example, the stomach is controlled by nerves that come from the mid back—the area between the shoulder blades. If there are Pressure Points between the shoulders that are blocking the nerve flow to the stomach, this could result in an upset stomach, ulcers or even chronic digestive problems. By treating these points with Pressure Point Therapy, the nerve flow once again opens up and the stomach problems can be reduced or even resolved.

It is interesting to observe that, while the person experiencing the stomach problems may or may not have pain between the shoulders, when these digestive Pressure Points are treated, it is often noticed that they are very tender.

The same holds true for headaches, back pain, and other conditions.

To Pressure Point or Medicate?

Pressure Point Therapy is not a cure all. It is simply a very effective technique that works more times than it doesn't. It doesn't take a rocket scientist to understand it and almost anyone can apply it on themselves and others.

The problem we are facing with our health care system is that there are too many rocket scientists out there. The complexity with which doctors view our bodies and the resultant mismanagement and unnecessary treatment is souring our taste and patience with the current medical profession.

FACT: It is reported that up to 80% of ALL SURGERIES ARE UNNECESSARY[1].

FACT: A large percentage of all emergency room admissions, 700,000 reported in one year, are due to a REACTION OF A PRESCRIPTION DRUG[2].

Pressure Point Therapy is not a substitute for the medical profession. It is just a rudimentary part of taking care of the body. The idea here is that if you apply Pressure Point Therapy and other healthy-life activities, you will move into the category of Health, not Sickness.

---

1 Lamb, Tom. "Back Surgery." *Centra*. Web. 21 Jun. 2012. <http://www.centrahealth.com/health-library/b/1304-back-surgery>.

2 "Adverse Drug Reactions Lead To 700,000 ER Visits Annually." *Drug Injury Watch*. 18 Oct 2006. Web. 21 Jun. 2012. <http://www.drug-injury.com/druginjurycom/2006/10/adverse_drug_ev.html>.

CHAPTER 2: RATING YOUR HEALTH—THE WELLNESS SCALE

The current definition of HEALTH in this country is truly twisted. Most people consider and define health as "not being sick." So when a person gets "sick" he runs to his doctor who treats him for his "condition."

The dictionary defines "health" as "having 100% function." This is far different than "not being sick."

The health of this country and other major parts of the world is in a dwindling spiral downward. Our health statistics continue to slide, even though we have such "great" high-tech medical care.

Who's to Blame

One can ask why and try to blame the medics, government and/or Big Pharma. I know I have! In investigating this, though, I found that the real reason why is our own gullibility and the fact we have blinders over our eyes. We have simply bought into the medical system too much and thus have given up our rights of common sense. And we ignore what we KNOW is right for ourselves.

USA Today ran an article on Alternative Health Care. The article cited that it was growing at an alarming rate, and that more people visited alternative practitioners than traditional doctors. Even so, medical "authorities" were "cautious" about these statistics, citing that these (alternative) treatments were "unproven" and "more studies were needed" to determine if they were effective. The medical profession, drug companies and government could be found guilty of one thing for sure: they promote that *their* way is the *only* way. They've gone out of their way to promote "Be wary of any alternatives." (They label most alternatives as "quack therapies.") They also withhold information from you regarding possible downfalls of their treatment procedures.

Plop Plop Fizz Fizz

When I was growing up watching TV, in the 1960's and '70's, drug companies began massive TV advertising campaigns which turned out to revolutionize their industry. At first their commercials were designed to bring about brand awareness. This was done through silly skits, effective jingles and humor.

Amongst the more memorable ads were "Excedrin Headache # ___," Pepto-Bismol commercials and Alka-Seltzer's "Plop Plop Fizz Fizz," and "I Can't Believe I Ate the Whole Thing."

Big Pharma was happy with the return on their investment and these commercials played on.

Part of the purpose in airing these drug commercials was to spread the message that it is normal to have headaches, monthly cramping, stomach problems and more. And the solutions were, of course, their drugs.

Today drug ads are completely out of control. During the Reagan Administration, direct-to-consumer drug advertising was made legal. Now, out of the goodness of their hearts, to "inform" us as a "public service," drug companies are spending billions of dollars to get into our heads.

These ads, which air constantly, are so expertly crafted, we begin to "self-diagnose" our problems. This has resulted in waves of patients storming into doctor's offices demanding to know if this "drug is right for me."

The cuteness of the 1970's "Plop Plop, Fizz Fizz" commercials has descended into vicious ads, complete with made-up diseases to boot. And of course, the FDA-approved drugs come to the rescue to treat these so-called disorders.

Normal conditions of life are now "serious diseases." Being a woman and having your period now has a half a dozen drugs to treat this "condition." Menopause is a psychiatric disorder. If you're having relationship problems, these are "symptoms" that you may be "depressed" or "bi-polar." Worse yet, your children are not "normal." They are drugging kids as young as six months old because they have temper-tantrums. The "disorders" ADD and ADHD (along with their addictive drug treatments) are more common in schools than chicken pox.

Common Sense Rules

Am I saying that all drug/medication use is unnecessary or bad? No. Just ask a diabetic what it is like to miss an insulin injection. I am not anti-drug.

But there are alternatives, and Pressure Point Therapy practiced on a regular basis will increase the health index of those receiving it.

Except in a health emergency situation, my rules for handling the body are:

1. Apply Pressure Point Therapy or Alternative treatment FIRST

2. Take drugs/medications SECOND

3. Surgery LAST

Now don't read into this and think that I am implying that Pressure Point Therapy, vitamins, chiropractic care, etc. is a cure-all or will revive the dead. It won't. If you have a health problem, you should still seek the advice of a health professional, such as a chiropractor or medical doctor.

But Pressure Point Therapy can be applied to anyone in almost any condition and it will help him feel better, relax and have better energy without any side effects.

You're Walking Around With It

Health officials have stated that in the last twenty to thirty years, the *type* of health problems people are experiencing has changed dramatically. People used to have diseases that resulted in long periods of bed rest, hospital stays, disabilities, etc. These were called Horizontal Diseases (because horizontal was the position one was in when confined to bed rest or a stay in a hospital).

The Horizontal Diseases included many infectious diseases such as polio, small pox, whooping cough, etc., and were so abundant that hospitals were filled to capacity as more were being built to handle the demand.

Today's health problems are very different. People have conditions that can't easily be shook, defined or treated. In fact, most are walking around with them, thus they are called Vertical Diseases. ("Vertical" denoting that a person is walking upright with their problems and "living with it.")

The Vertical Diseases have ousted Horizontal Diseases and are now the commonplace. Some of these include headaches, PMS, chronic fatigue syndrome, back pains, TMJ (jaw pain), carpal tunnel syndrome (wrist pain), fibromyalgia (pain anywhere and everywhere in the body), metabolic syndrome (weight gain and pre-diabetes) and many more.

The Vertical Diseases have nearly emptied hospitals. Hospitals have closed, merged or have become specialized, such as birth centers.

Vertical Diseases generally DO NOT RESPOND TO DRUG THERAPIES, or "modern medicine" as we know it. I can't tell you how many patients I have seen who have told me that they took themselves off of a medication because it didn't work. It made them sicker, more tired or doped-up. Or it simply covered up a symptom.

Pressure Point Therapy works FANTASTICALLY on these Vertical Diseases. You will hear raves of how great a person feels even after one treatment. As you practice this technique and become confident, you will find that YOU can change many conditions on yourself, family and friends.

"I Think It's Due to Stress"

The medical profession is truly frustrated with the Vertical Diseases. After many failures with a multitude of drugs, doctors will often go that *extra step* and tell you that your problems are "due to stress" and that it is "all in your head." Or "you're depressed."

To exemplify this point, I was in the studio recording a radio show for Pressure Point Therapy. At the break, the recording engineer, who had been listening to my show, said she was interested in the technique because she had carpal tunnel syndrome (wrist pain). Being on the soundboard all day, she over-used her wrist and hand.

She told me she went to her medical doctor for the problem. I was curious as to how he would treat her, so I asked her what he did for her.

"He prescribed an anti-depressant."
"What?"

Well, she had been in a bad relationship and was working too much and the doctor thought she was depressed...

How a wrist problem and anti-depressants go together, I'll never know.

This example sheds light on how pill-happy doctors have become and how the public has seemingly bought into it.

Just as a note, anti-depressant usage has grown to the point that one out of four women in this country are now on anti-depressants. There is also a growing problem of prescription drugs being prescribed "off-label" (not for their intended use, such as this example above). I've seen statistics that prescription medicine abuse is now greater than illegal drug use in teenagers. Also, over 90,000 deaths, just in the US, occur each year due to reactions to these drugs.

So what is it that we are looking for? The risk/reward ratio of modern medicine is getting trickier at best.

We want to feel relaxed, we want to be ourselves and have lots of health and energy.

Pressure Point Therapy helps a person relax. It helps the nerves function. If one is under stress, many times Pressure Point Therapy will help "reset" the body. For those of you who are computer savvy, it is like Control-Alt-Delete (keys on a computer for rebooting the computer or in this example, the body).

The Wellness Scale

So where is this leading? It is important to understand the application of the Pressure Point Therapy technique, and you will for sure learn this as you read on.

But equally important is to grasp the purpose for applying the technique: what is the end-result, what do you want to accomplish?

I have created the Wellness Scale to help you and your family clarify your own health goals.

The Wellness Scale is a chart that helps define exact states of health (or sickness) so you can determine your own health status or the health of others. It gives you a base-line of where you're at and shows you the heights of true health.

Just like a person who is on a diet and keeps a graph or chart of their weight loss, the Wellness Scale allows you to plot your changes as you go from lower to higher states of health.

Wellness Scale Procedure

Read over the chart and the characteristics of each level. Then plot your own health on the chart before you start receiving Pressure Point Therapy. Repeat after two to four weeks. Like many people who are applying this technique and other health-related activities, you'll find your level rising.

After working with the human body for over thirty years, I have made an interesting observation: the body is VERY appreciative for any HEALTH measures you send in its direction. In fact, a little health goes a long way.

Pressure Point Therapy seems to be the forgotten or lost key that unlocks and opens the door to wellness. Through it you can erase what seems to be life-long aches and pains, low energy and other unwanted conditions. As stated earlier in this book, Pressure Point Therapy is a lost art now recovered. Most people love this technique because their conditions change so quickly, treatment to treatment.

The Wellness Scale is another tool that you can use to not only change your body, but also your viewpoint about health.

Setting Goals

It would be apparent that most people would want to be at the top of the Wellness Scale. But reality has it where one can be in the middle or even near the bottom of the scale. So it is important to set a realistic goal for yourself and then use this technique to achieve it.

A person who had just fractured his leg may have a goal to play sports again. But this would take a minimum of four to six weeks so the body has time to heal. If you are suffering from some unwanted pain or condition, have as your first goal, feeling less pain. I used to tell patients at the clinic who went from severe, acute pain to being "stiff all over" that this is an improvement! Why? They are going from pain to stiffness! A true marker of getting better!

The point is, make mental (or actual) notes on your improvement(s) by utilizing Pressure Point Therapy. You may be pleasantly surprised how much better you are feeling!

And remember, don't stop just because you are feeling better. There is a lot of health ahead of you on the Wellness Scale!

THE WELLNESS SCALE

	Condition	Characteristics	
	Condition	*Characteristics*	*Health Care*
100	100% Function	Body is running perfectly and has longevity.	
90	Cell Protection	Body recognizes abnormal cells and destroys them, keeping cell integrity.	
80	Cell Rejuvination	Old cells are replaced with young new cells, leading to anti-aging or slowed aging.	
70	Immune Function	Person doesn't get sick very often, if at all. Recovers quickly if does.	
60	High Energy	Person has an abundance of energy and regenerates well after a good night's sleep.	
50	No Symptoms	Dangerous state. Most people consider this to be "health." Simply an absence of symptoms.	
40	Low Energy/Fatigue	Always feel tired. Tends to do caffeine, sugar etc. If the body stays this way, it drops to 30.	
30	Pain/Sickness/Run-down	Always getting sick or complaining. Seeks medical help frequently. Often on medications.	
20	Diagnosed Condition	Has a "disease" or "condition." Is a definite medical case.	
10	Serious Condition	Very advanced condition. Poor prognosis. May be terminal. Surgery often.	
0	Death	No function.	

Sick Care

Wellness Scale: Facts and Figures

Here are some other interesting notes regarding the Wellness Scale:

- From around 35 down to 0 on the Wellness Scale, the medical profession awaits your arrival. *Sickness* is where your doctor's attention is focused. And he is firmly fixed in "drugging it" or "cutting it out." This is why many traditional doctors cannot fathom how or why Pressure Point Therapy works (or any other valid Alternative Health technique). They could be very skeptical of it (and thus promote their "expert" opinion). Medical procedures here include the dispensing of prescription drugs (usually multiple prescriptions; the average person in the US is on several "meds"), lots of medical tests (and if you have good insurance, the more tests you will receive), surgeries, being told, "You have to live with it," etc.

- When a person is at 30 Pain/Sickness/Rundown and he goes to the doctor, the doctor usually prescribes a medication. The medication will often times mask the pain/symptom so the person does not feel the symptom. This now temporarily (and artificially) raises the person on the scale to 40 Low Energy/Fatigue. It is a commonly known fact that most medications have side effects of zapping a person's energy, resulting in drowsiness and being tired, or 40 Low Energy/Fatigue on the Wellness Scale.

- You can be stuck between 30 Pain/Sickness/Rundown and 40 Low Energy/Fatigue. When a person is wiped out all of the time (at 40 Low Energy/Fatigue), his immune system lowers and he becomes susceptible to getting sick. The person then tends to fall down on the scale back to the area of 30 Pain/Sickness/Rundown. This is the person who gets sick over and over again. Eventually the person wears down to 20 Diagnosed Condition, where a named disease or disorder has labeled the condition.

- One of the most dangerous places to be is at 50 No Symptoms. A person here marvels at waking up with no pain, not having a headache and not being sick. This is dangerous because most people feel this is the *best* place they could be. Many serious or even fatal conditions have NO SYMPTOMS connected to them. There are, of course, higher states of health.

- At 60 High Energy, true Health Care begins. We know that Health = Function. Here we find a person beginning to function much better. When Pressure Point Therapy is applied, it helps reduce the stress along the nerves. As the nerve blockages release, the nerve begins to function better. The body's energy can then flow throughout the body. The result: having High Energy consistently, without effort, caffeine or other artificial means.

- 70, 80 and 90 on the Wellness Scale represent very high states of health. The body's immune system is working, taking out bacteria, viruses, fungi and abnormal or damaged cells, such as cancer and arthritis type cells.

- At these higher states, a person "ages" slower too. Every three to four months the body replaces all of the cells with new ones. "Aging" could be considered as having substandard replacement cells. If your body is replacing your cells with damaged or weakened cells, you begin to feel "age."

At higher levels of health, the body can recognize if a cell is a "dud" and uses the power of the immune system to remove it so it doesn't multiply and create a condition. For your information, the immune system is controlled by the nervous system in the body.

- When a person is at 70 Immune Function, he generally does not get sick. How many people do you know that "get everything"? When at 70, if a person does get sick, he bounces back quickly.

- One of the important attributes that will be found in people who are above 50 is that the person does not have attention on his body. People below 50 constantly know that they are hurting or not feeling well; their body is being a problem.

Pressure Point Therapy is a valuable tool in helping you and your family increase your positions on the Wellness Scale. Let's move on now to applying Pressure Point Therapy.

CHAPTER 3: APPLYING PRESSURE POINT THERAPY

Applying Pressure Point Therapy is easy. It can be done to oneself but is best performed by another. There are devices available to help you reach areas—like your back—if you are using Pressure Point Therapy on yourself. (See "Chapter 10: Do-It-Yourself Pressure Point Massagers and Devices.")

Traditional Pressure Point Therapy involves using your hands, specifically your thumbs and fingers, to place pressure over various points on the body. There are several Pressure Point charts in Part II of this book that are categorized by condition. Once the Pressure Points are found using these charts, you simply follow the instructions on the charts as to where to start, where to go next, etc.

Firm pressure is applied to the point until the stress held in the Pressure Point is "released." The release occurs when the recipient states that there is less pain or sensation over the Pressure Point.

Or, once you become proficient, you can actually *feel* the Pressure Point release. It can be subtle. To many if feels like air has been released from a tire. It is common for Pressure Point Therapists (those who have read and practiced the techniques from this book) to actually feel the area of the Pressure Point relax, right under their finger tips. The first few times this happens you and your recipient can hardly believe it. But it is really occurring!

Communication

Communication is important, especially getting feedback from your recipient. Ask questions such as "Do you feel this point?" or "Has the pain here lessened at all?"

You should not use the treatment time to chat, chatter or talk about the day or family. A Pressure Point Therapy treatment is not like getting your hair done. You are helping your recipient by finding and treating Pressure Points. Other than getting feedback about using the correct amount of pressure, being on the exact spot or whether or not the Pressure Point has released, you should keep the conversation to a minimum. The purpose is to have the recipient get relief and relax, after all.

Technique

It is best to have the recipient lying face down comfortably or sitting. If the recipient is lying down, it is OK to have pillows available to prop up parts of the body. A person can lay down anywhere: a bed, couch or even the floor, on a rug or on towels. You can also purchase a massage table if you're getting into the technique. The price has really come down on these and they are nice to have. Comfort is the main idea here. Most of the Pressure Points are on the back, but some are on the front of the body, arms, legs and head.

The correct Pressure Point chart should be selected based on the complaints of the individual or based on the desired results.

(Pressure Point Therapy can be utilized daily for general body toning and increased energy—one doesn't have to have a problem. See the chart "General Pressure Points for Greater Vitality and Energy" in Part II of this book.)

Each Pressure Point chart will instruct you which point to treat and in what order.

Too Little, Too Much

There is a rule for the correct amount of pressure to be used in doing this technique: you need to apply enough pressure to the Pressure Point so it can be felt by the recipient. "Felt" here means there is usually some point-tenderness or actual pain over the area. It should not be so uncomfortable to the point where the recipient is squirming or wincing. Too little pressure, on the other hand, doesn't release the energy from the point. Way too much pressure causes the recipient to tighten up, resulting in the person actually holding *more* pressure. There is a "just-right" amount and practicing will make perfect.

Most people have a tendency to go too light. Don't be afraid to "get in there." Watch the recipient's body language and responses. If you end up with the *Pressure Point Therapy DVD* I demonstrate how to apply Pressure Point Therapy very specifically. (You can order the DVD by visiting www.pressurepointtherapy.com.)

My Pressure Point "grip" is quite firm. Again, you don't want to be so firm as to shock someone. Once you find the Pressure Point, you can gradually increase the pressure. It is a trial-and-error thing. Individuals have their own sensitivity threshold and you have to adjust the pressure accordingly.

Sometimes a person will be in acute pain (hurts to move, etc.). It could be that the person's back is out or possibly strained from a workout. Be gentle enough so you don't shock the body, but firm enough to get the results. Also, the Pressure Points will lighten up after several passes, so you might have to go over the chart two or three times before the tension is removed from the Pressure Points.

Breathe!

If you get on Pressure Points that are uncomfortable or painful, have the recipient breathe out (exhale) while you press down on the point. This is very important. Breathing out will help tremendously in releasing the Pressure Point. This is again covered in the *Pressure Point Therapy DVD*. This will also help relieve the pain.

The treatment motion is slow and intent. Don't rush it. Many body pressures are caused by the fast-paced world in which we operate.

One treats the first Pressure Point on the chart, lets up, goes to the second set of points, lets up, then goes to the third set, and so on. The person treating also makes mental notes of where the sorest points are. He/she will be going back to do more work on them.

The technique is to contact the Pressure Points with firm pressure and press down slowly until the point has "nowhere to go" and is covered by the thumb or finger. This extreme position is held for a moment or two (up to ten to fifteen seconds for real sore Pressure Points). Then the pressure is let up and the next point is contacted.

If one has a very sore Pressure Point do not try to handle it in one pass. Go to other points and work on them, then revisit the painful one. Have the recipient use his breathing to help release the point, applying more pressure as the recipient exhales.

Many times, you will need to remind your recipient to breathe, as there is a tendency for a person to hold hig breath as you are applying pressure. And you may have to lighten up your contact. Be in communication with your recipient and watch his body language.

Repeating the pattern of points can be done two to three times, and the treatment itself usually lasts four to five minutes or longer. Some people will not want you to stop!

Results

The recipient will feel relaxed, have greater energy and have a sense of relief from the problems he was experiencing. If working with a child or even an infant, they may be resting quietly when complete.

Don't leave a situation unresolved or a Pressure Point unreleased. You may have to take a rest for ten to thirty minutes and treat the person again. The goal is having the recipient feel better and having him know that his condition is changing.

CHAPTER 4: HOW TO FIND PRESSURE POINTS

What do Pressure Points feel like? Well, this depends on whether you are applying the treatment or receiving it!

From the Pressure Point Therapist's point of view, a Pressure Point may feel like a small knot or even like a marble.

The Pressure Points can be close to the surface or they may be deeper. When the points are deeper, it may take more "oomph" to treat them. Again, you need to watch the recipient's indicators so you don't go too hard.

Remember, one of the primary goals of Pressure Point Therapy is to RELAX the body. Most Pressure Points are connected to nerves and nerves are very sensitive indeed.

That's The Spot!

An *active* Pressure Point (one that requires you to hold the spot until the tenderness goes away), always has a sensation associated with it when you push on it. This, of course, is from the recipient's point of view. The sensation can range from a deep burning pain to a slight area of discomfort to a ticklish feeling.

If you encounter a spot that tickles the recipient, the correct treatment technique is to gradually increase pressure on the Pressure Point until the recipient senses more of a pain feeling than a tickle sensation. The recipient will then indicate to you that the point hurts, burns, etc.

In Part II of this book you will find individual Pressure Point charts for many conditions. These charts will show you where the Pressure Points are and the patterns for treating them. As you run through the points when treating someone, you will find some of the Pressure Points will not have sensations associated with them. These points are therefore not active. It is still OK to treat these Pressure Points as part of your pattern, but you will spend more time on the active or sore points.

Hot Spots

We are looking for active Pressure Points. During your first pass using a Pressure Point chart as the "map," you are scouting for the sore ones. You will then stop at the sore or active point and release it, per the instructions above. Several passes may be needed. You generally will work them out until the pain lessens or disappears completely.

If the Pressure Point doesn't resolve, don't try to treat it all at once. Make note of its location and go back later and treat it again.

Some people have been carrying this stress around for a lifetime. You don't have to "erase it" all in one treatment period.

Where Are They?

Most of the Pressure Points are located on the back. Why? Because Pressure Points follow the nerve pathways on the body and 80% of all nerves are located in the back.

Your back contains the spine, spinal nerves and muscles. The spine consists of twenty-four or twenty-five movable bones called vertebrae. For each vertebra, there are two main nerves that exit through the sides of the bone, one to the left and one to the right. These nerves are called the spinal nerves. The spinal nerves continue to branch out through the body and supply the nerve energy to all of the organs, glands, bones and muscles.

The main Pressure Point "highway" is located about *1" to either side of the center of the spine*. This is where the major nerve blockages occur which can shut down a person's energy.

Lighten Up

At this point you might be grumbling to yourself, "Geez, I though this was going to be easy/now there is (yuck) anatomy/what if I don't find the point exactly or hit the wrong point and ... and ..."

Don't worry. You will be getting more instruction as the book goes on, and I did promise you that Pressure Point Therapy *is* easy to learn and apply.

Also, it doesn't hurt if you do not treat the Pressure Point exactly. Any Pressure Point Therapy is better than none. Practice will make perfect.

CHAPTER 5: PRESSURE POINTS—HOW TO TREAT

The treatment of Pressure Points is simple. It consists of applying pressure to the point until it "releases" or lessens in intensity.

The technique for doing this is to apply thumb or finger pressure over the Pressure Point. Begin lightly and then gradually increase the amount of pressure you are using. If you have sore or arthritic hands, you can be assisted by a number of hand-held Pressure Knobbers. See "Chapter 10: Do-It-Yourself Pressure Point Massagers and Devices."

If you are using a Pressure Pointer on yourself, the procedure is basically the same, going point to point and spending more time with the active ones.

Breathe Out—Push Down

It works best if you can push down on a Pressure Point while the recipient is exhaling. This is especially useful when you are working on the back and when you encounter a real painful Pressure Point.

Instruct the recipient to breathe out as you are pressing down or into the Pressure Point. This doesn't have to be labored breathing. Just have the recipient use his normal expiration.

When the recipient breathes in, you relax your contact slightly. When he breathes out, you push into the Pressure Point a little deeper. And repeat.

When you come across a very sore Pressure Point, you can have the recipient take deeper breaths as you work out the point deeper.

Most of the time, however, you will have the recipient just breathe normally. Use this rhythm-breathing technique in the event you're working on real sore points and they are stubborn in releasing.

Treating Very Sore Pressure Points

You will come across very sore Pressure Points where the recipient will flinch with pain. Now you know that you have a very "good" spot, an area where the nerve energy has been blocked and is concentrated around the nerve (and therefore the very tender Pressure Point).

Prior to treating this spot, you will need to know if the recipient had any kind of injury that would have bruised the area or resulted in a torn muscle, broken bone, etc. Such can be a from a fall or car accident. We obviously do NOT treat bruised tissues, areas of broken bone, recent surgeries or infections. Common sense has to be part of your application of Pressure Point Therapy.

Also, if you ever have any questions or anything medical comes up, be sure to consult your doctor before beginning Pressure Point treatments. See more about this in "Chapter 9: Precautions."

Under normal circumstances (which is 99.99% of the time), when you encounter a real sore one, first acknowledge to your recipient that you have found an active Pressure Point. Let them know that this is what you're looking for and that you will be treating the Pressure Point to release it.

You will need to begin with a more gentle touch. Gradually increase the amount of pressure over the Pressure Point, working with the recipient's breathing as above. Repeat the downward pressure over the Pressure Point, working with the exhale as you push down. It may take three to four complete breathing cycles (in & out breaths) to fully release this Pressure Point.

If your recipient is in a lot of pain, let's say lower back pain, have them ice the area first with an ice pack wrapped in a towel. After twenty minutes or so treat the person with the correct Pressure Point Therapy Chart, located in Part II of this book.

Releasing a Pressure Point

As the Pressure Point releases or loosens up, there are certain things you (as the Pressure Point Therapist) will be able to feel:

You may first feel the area tightening up slightly. This will begin to loosen as you continue to apply pressure.

You next may feel the most "gosh darn" thing: the Pressure Point begins to "melt" under your finger or thumb. It feels like the point is "dissolving," right then and there! What you are actually feeling is the reduction of the muscle spasm that is blocking the nerve.

You may also feel an intense heat reaction as the Pressure Point releases. This again is a sign that the energy is once again flowing through the area. The heat may extend one or two hand lengths. Have the recipient or other observers feel the area with their hands if possible. They will be able to for sure feel the difference.

It may take five to six rounds of finger/thumb pressure over the Pressure Point with the breathing before it releases. If it doesn't release after ten to twenty seconds or so, go on and make note of this Pressure Point. Additional treatment over this area may be needed at a later time.

Quick Fix

Beware of the Quick Fix Syndrome. This is what has led to the downfall of modern health in our society—people want to feel good now, at any expense. Pressure Point Therapy is not a drug. It may take several treatments before a person begins to realize the benefits of the therapy.

I know one doctor who practices Alternative Health Care who will not even accept a patient unless he commits to a two-month program, where he is treated three times a week. Although this is extreme, it demonstrates the fact that Pressure Point Therapy may take time to produce results.

Remember, good natural healing can take time!

You may also experience miraculous, fast results as well.

It often takes years for a person to destroy his body. Or he may have had a condition for years. Be persistent and encourage your recipients to be patient as well.

Well Done

Don't do too much in a Pressure Point Therapy treatment. Unlike a massage, Pressure Point Therapy works directly with the nerve channels in the body. This means that the treatments are "concentrated." You get a lot more bang for your buck with Pressure Point Therapy. A typical Pressure Point Therapy treatment may last for five to fifteen minutes. Some can go longer.

The general rule is try to handle one or, at the most, two problems or problem-areas per treatment. Trying to treat every condition a person has in one treatment can result in an "over-done" phenomena. The person will have gone past the point where it was very relaxing and beneficial. Take it one step at a time.

Feeling Sore After Treatment

A person may tighten up slightly or feel "knocked out" after a Pressure Point Treatment. This is a normal reaction, especially at first. There are toxins and wastes in the body that are held into the muscles surrounding Pressure Points. These toxins can be released into the system (to be processed out) when the Pressure Points are treated. This is no concern. An hour of rest or a good night's sleep will help. It is similar to beginning a workout and feeling sore afterwards.

You should also instruct your recipient to drink more water following his treatments. This will help minimize any tightness or tiredness as the water flushes the toxins through the body. Having shorter treatment sessions will also minimize any reactions.

Get the Correct Pressure

The question comes up of how much pressure to use when treating a Pressure Point. Using too soft of a touch does not get to the root of the Pressure Point. Going too hard is both uncomfortable and can upset or hurt the recipient. It takes practice to get the correct pressure applied. The recipient should be able to "feel" an active Pressure Point when you are treating it, but the sensation should not be unbearable.

Most people who learn Pressure Point Therapy will at first be too gentle. Practice "getting in there" with an adult, one who is in good shape. You will soon learn what is acceptable and what is too much or too little.

Being in good communication with your recipient is key—watching his facial expressions and body language. Squirming or arms and legs flying are indications of too much pressure. Get feedback from him, asking if the amount of pressure you are using is OK. He will be able to tell you if it is too little or too much.

Your recipients may also be able to guide you to the point. "Just down and to the right," is a common response from your recipient. But don't count on this alone, as the sensory nerves which point out where you're touching can be poor, especially on the back.

If the recipient is giving you no reaction, or you get a comment like "This isn't doing anything," it can be an indicator that you're using too little pressure. The person should feel the treatment and know that the Pressure Points which were there have diminished in pain.

Tired Hands

You will find that your hands, fingers, thumbs and wrists will tend to get tired very quickly (especially to begin with) when you are treating with Pressure Point Therapy. This is normal. You are allowed to and should momentarily rest your hands during treatment. Your hands, fingers, thumbs and wrists will build up as you continue to apply the technique. Check out "Chapter 10: Do-It-Yourself Pressure Point Massagers" for different tools, such as hand-held knobbers, to help assist you.

Your body positioning is also important. If you use only your hands to treat the points, you'll tire. Position your body over your arms, so when you find an active Pressure Point, you can use some of your body weight to treat the area. Also make sure *you* are comfortable. You don't want to get cramped up doing a treatment!

CHAPTER 6: BODY LANDMARKS

There are certain landmarks that you will need to know so you can easily cross-reference the Pressure Point Charts with the body. Study the following Landmark Chart and then find these landmarks on a real person.

BODY LANDMARKS

- SINUS POINTS
- JAW POINTS
- COLLARBONE AREA
- CHEST BONE (STERNUM)
- PMS POINTS (SIDE OF LEG)
- BASE OF THE SKULL
- PRESSURE POINT 'ALLEY'
- DIMPLE IN THE GLUTEUS AREA

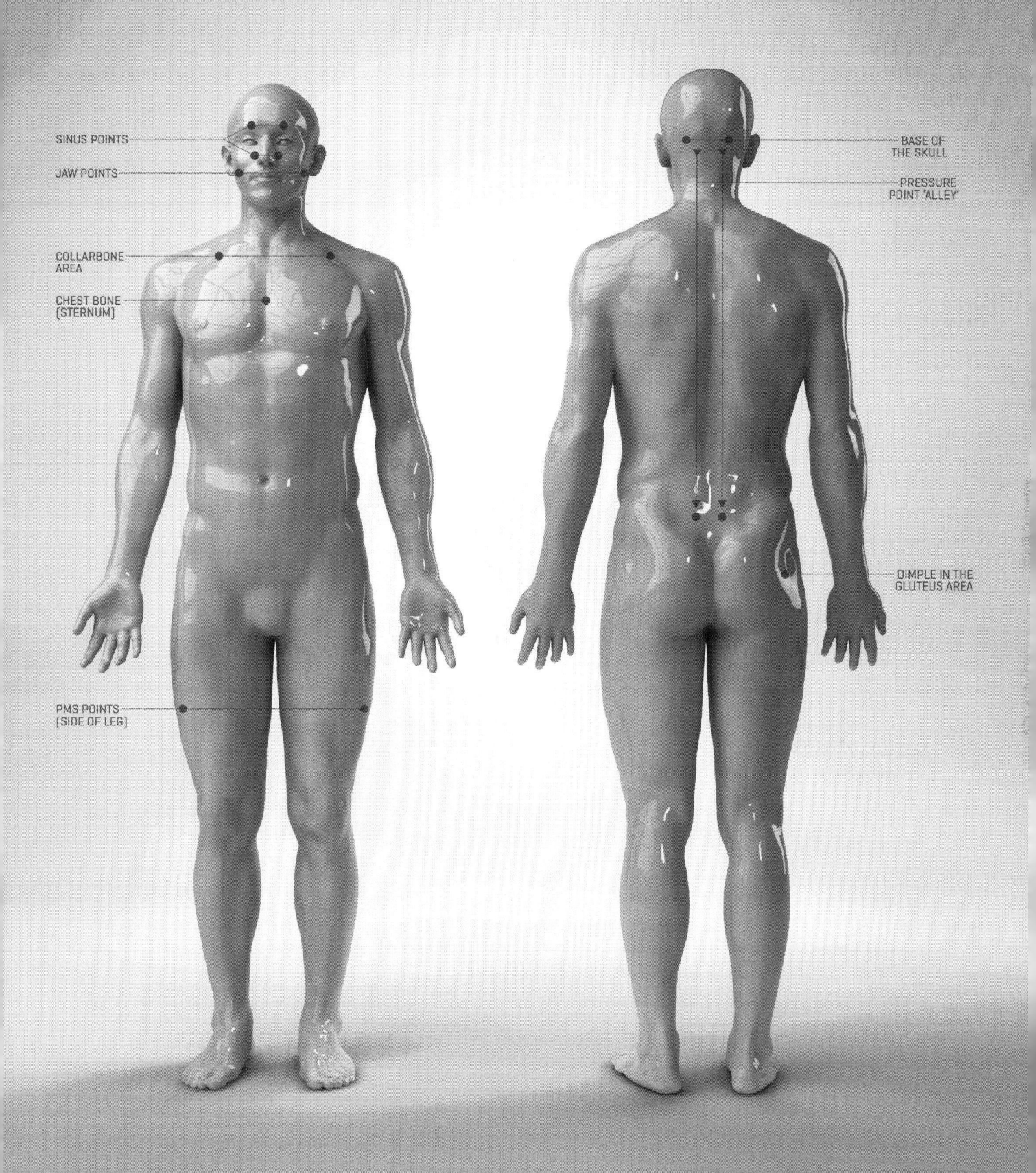

CHAPTER 7: THE ABC'S OF APPLYING PRESSURE POINT THERAPY

You are now ready to begin practicing. The key here is to go slow, get the feel for Pressure Points and practice some more. I have been treating patients as a doctor for thirty years and they still call it "practice."

Use the chart "General Pressure Points for Greater Energy and Vitality" located in Part II as your practice chart.

Where to Apply Pressure Point Therapy

You do not need any special equipment or tables to apply Pressure Point Therapy. It can be done on a couch, bed or, as I prefer, on the floor. A massage table is also useful, especially the portable types if you are going to be doing a lot of treatment. Stores like Costco or Amazon.com carry portable massage tables and they are quite reasonably priced.

Environment is also very important. The treatment space should have the following qualities: it should be warm, private, quiet as possible, and without distractions such as children or pets. The recipient should lie on a blanket, towel or carpeting if on the floor. You can have a pillow and a glass of water handy. Of course you should have this Pressure Point Therapy book nearby, so you can reference the Pressure Point Therapy Charts.

Oh yes, cell phones off? For sure!

What should I Wear?

The recipient should wear loose clothes if possible. A tee shirt or blouse works well, as you can feel the points through the clothing. It is not necessary to be treated on the bare skin or to be naked. I do not advise this.

The person treating should also wear loose clothes and be in a comfortable position. Don't strain your body by bending over, etc. It is easy to hurt yourself or get cramped up.

For example, if you are treating someone on a bed, instead of bending over the bed, make some room for you to sit or kneel on the bed next to your recipient. Both you and your recipient have to be comfortable.

How to Begin

First off, you should go over the Landmark Chart and practice finding these areas on another person. The more you can get used to feeling with you hands, the better off you'll be. If you have the *Pressure Point Therapy DVD,* watch this, preferably with another. You'll be able to practice and do demonstrations on each other while playing the DVD.

Practice on your family or friends. Be patient and keep it simple. Start with the "General Pressure Points for Greater Energy and Vitality" chart. Ideally, you would treat someone and then have them treat you. You will become one hundred times better if you can receive Pressure Point Therapy as well as give it.

Pressure Point Therapy on the Couch

Begin a ritual of applying Pressure Point Therapy on each other if you are in a relationship. Many couples are so busy in life, they don't get "quality" time together.

When you're watching TV, it is easy to reach over to your spouse and begin working on him/her. It is quite relaxing too.

If you're someone who is looking to change your lifestyle and become healthier, substitute eating junk food or having that drink after work "to relax" and try Pressure Point Therapy instead. Get yourself and your friend or significant other energized by applying five to ten minutes of Pressure Point Therapy.

Pressure Point and Children

One of the greatest applications of Pressure Point Therapy is with children. I could write an entire book on how Pressure Point Therapy works with children. I've used it extensively. With my own family, everyone scores it a "10."

Keeping a child's nerves functioning properly also improves his immune system. Immunity is directly connected to the nervous system. When our child was growing up, we had to use antibiotics only once or twice. You'll find ear infections, coughs, digestive problems and many other conditions respond to Pressure Point Therapy.

I've also had great success with Attention Deficit, autism and other childhood problems. You can visit my web site, drpinkus.com or my Facebook site, facebook.com/drpinkus for more detailed information about this.

It is interesting that in other parts of the world, a mother massaging her child is part of her daily routine. I've seen works on this and it is fascinating.

Children respond quickly to Pressure Point Therapy because they don't have long patterns built up in their bodies. I've used it on infants (very light touch) and on children who couldn't get to sleep.

Remember, the nervous system controls everything in the body. Once you can begin to effectively influence the nerves, the person goes up the Wellness Scale.

Treatment Procedure

First, locate the proper chart for the problem you are working on. The Pressure Point Therapy Charts in Part II of this book are categorized according to condition. If there isn't a specific chart for the problem you are seeking to treat, use the chart closest to the problem.

For example, if you're treating an ear ache, use the "Pressure Points for Sinuses, Allergies, Head Colds and Congestion" chart. If you're treating Tennis Elbow, use the "Pressure Points for Hand, Wrist and Elbow Pain" chart.

Once you have the appropriate chart, follow the instructions on the chart and go through the pattern once with your recipient. Then repeat the pattern. Having made mental notes on the sore or active Pressure Points, go back and treat the individual points you found to be the sorest. Treat each point until your recipient is feeling less pain or until the pain goes away. If the points remain sore, take note of their location and treat them again at another time.

CHAPTER 8: FREQUENCY OF TREATMENT

Pressure Point Therapy can be performed several times a day if need be. You have to be realistic with how much you can give or take. Many people find Pressure Point Therapy so relaxing or invigorating that they love to receive it daily.

If you are higher on the Wellness Scale, you can have treatments whenever you wish. At least one time per week is desirable and therapeutic. If you are treating a condition, such as back pain, you should receive treatments a minimum of three times per week.

If you are having chronic fatigue, try receiving Pressure Point Therapy instead of coffee in the morning. Or if you are having trouble relaxing, getting a Pressure Point Therapy treatment in the evening can do wonders and help you get a good night sleep.

For acute or severe conditions, receiving treatment daily or even several times per day is beneficial. In severe conditions or if you have questions, be sure to seek advice from your chiropractor or doctor. Remember, Pressure Point Therapy is not a cure-all, and it is unwise to take undue risks with your health or that of another.

As a note, giving Pressure Point Therapy is as important as receiving it—maybe more important. Your ability to help another is one of man's greatest virtues.

CHAPTER 9: PRECAUTIONS

If any condition you are trying to treat persists or gets worse, you need to consult a doctor. Pressure Point Therapy is not a substitute for medical or chiropractic care. In many instances, it is a benefit along with these other treatments. But this book is not meant to replace a chiropractic treatment, if called for, or a medical doctor's opinion or professional advice.

Never apply Pressure Point Therapy on open sores or wounds or infected areas. Do not apply Pressure Point Therapy to broken bones or areas of intense swelling. If a person has a severe medical condition, do not apply Pressure Point Therapy without permission first from his/her doctor. Always be mindful of what you are doing.

With pregnant mothers, avoid any pressure over the top or sides of the belly. Pregnant mothers should not lie on their stomachs after the third month. Lying on the side is OK.

On people who have circulatory problems, such as arteriosclerosis, diabetes, blood clots, stroke history etc., do not apply pressure to the leg areas.

Never mix Pressure Point Therapy with any sexual activities. Pressure Point Therapy is not a *sensual* activity. It is a *healing* activity and it is your responsibility to be professional while applying and receiving Pressure Point Therapy.

Pressure Point Therapy can be applied on children and infants, but only with a great reduction in pressure. On infants or younger children the amount of pressure I use is as much as putting a stamp on an envelope. Just the weight of your index finger alone is enough.

On older bodies, senior citizens, also reduce the pressure applied. As a general rule, always be much more gentle in your touch with children, elderly people and persons recovering from some illness or surgery.

NEVER attempt to adjust, manipulate or "crack" any person's spine or any other part of his/her body. NEVER try to mimic your chiropractor in using this technique. Chiropractors and osteopaths receive training for years to learn how to adjust the spine and it could be very dangerous to attempt to do so yourself.

Questions

If you have any questions at all regarding who can receive Pressure Point Therapy, consult your chiropractor or medical doctor.

Remember, Pressure Point Therapy is not a cure-all and has never been promoted as such. You will be very pleased with what it can do, but do not attempt to BE a doctor just because you know this technique. You can ask questions or leave comments at facebook.com/drpinkus.

CHAPTER 10: DO-IT-YOURSELF PRESSURE POINT MASSAGERS AND DEVICES

My Ideal Notion

In the first edition of this book, I had the notion that once one learned Pressure Point Therapy, he would recruit his spouse, child, significant other or even co-worker to also learn the technique and then begin doing exchanges on each other. A fairly high percentage did exactly that.

But then there are those who can only "receive," for whatever reason. And a number of people lived alone. So I set off to find what I call a "Pressure Pointer" or a device one could use on himself to treat his own Pressure Points.

Contortion Specialists?

Being that many of the Pressure Points are located on one's back, unless one was a performer for Cirque du Soleil, it would be improbable that one could be limber enough to reach behind to treat these points.

So as humans tend to find solutions to their problems, I have found a number of great devices that will do the trick. Many of these are made from very high-density materials, like fiberglass, heavy plastics or aluminum, which are needed to treat the Pressure Points with the correct force and be sturdy enough to hold up over time.

There's a Hook to the Design…

The best Pressure Pointers are designed so one could easily reach over his shoulder or around to the back to "hook" the Pressure Point and treat it. So the devices I use are mostly "C-shaped" and some are "S-shaped." They are also large enough to get the job done.

The best way to get your own hands on one of my Pressure Pointers is to visit one of my web sites. You can check these out at the following:

pressurepointtherapy.com

facebook.com/drpinkus

drpinkus.com

By the way, I am using these web sites as information portals. When you visit these sites you can sign up for free updates, webinars, and my radio and TV appearances. You can also ask me questions, especially on Facebook.

The procedure for connecting up with me on Facebook, at least at the time of printing, is to "Like" my Facebook page, which puts you in the mix to send and receive communications from me. (Facebook changes their procedures and policies like the wind so this could change...)

How to Use a Pressure Pointer on Yourself

The procedure for using a Pressure Pointer on yourself is almost identical to treating another:

1. Have this book by your side, opened to the appropriate chart for the condition you want to treat.
2. You should be in a comfortable position, in a chair is usually best.
3. Using the Pressure Pointer, reach behind you and find the first Pressure Point from the chart you are using. Pull the Pressure Pointer *forward* to increase the pressure on the point.
4. If it is an Active Pressure Point, then hold the pressure over the spot for ten to fifteen seconds or until the pain starts to lighten up or relieve itself altogether.
5. Then go to the next Pressure Point on the chart and continue. Spend time with the most Active Pressure Points.
6. Once you have gone through the chart, repeat as necessary or until you feel good.

Applying Pressure Point Therapy—Almost Anywhere at Anytime

You are going to get addicted to this technique, I promise. This isn't so terrible, considering all of the bad stuff out there one could get addicted to!

I have a number of users who have acquired several Pressure Pointers. They leave one by the couch and treat their Pressure Points while watching TV. They have one by their bed and do a treatment before going to sleep or upon arising.

Then there are those who have an extra Pressure Pointer at work, which is a great stress-buster. When under stress you pull out your Pressure Pointer and go to town. Low energy, neck pain, back stiffness— all gone in five minutes or less!

You're Not Fit While You Sit

"I'll just sit myself down and relax."

NOT.

Sitting, according to researchers, is the most STRESSFUL position your body can be in. Testing confirmed that while sitting, the discs in the lower back were beyond their "breaking" point. In other words, sitting overloads the lower back more than the discs, muscles and ligaments were meant to take.

Besides this, we're sitting more than ever before, averaging 9.3 hours per day. We sleep 7.7 hours per day on average, in comparison. So if you have to sit because you're at work or on the computer, get up often. And do your Pressure Point Therapy too, right at your desk, work-station or couch.

One of the reasons sitting is so detrimental to your health is that sitting shuts off much of the electrical activity going into your legs. We know that applying Pressure Point Therapy increases energy throughout the entire body, including the legs.

So having a Pressure Pointer at work and at home can help reverse the downfalls of sitting.

Hand Knobbers

Some people think my hands are so strong that I could open a can of soup without a can opener. Well this is not quite true, but as you do Pressure Point Therapy your strength will greatly improve, especially in your arms and hands.

As your hands are very sensitive and "perceptive," it is best to use your hands whenever possible. There are, however, a few good tools that are helpful if you don't have the strength or endurance, or if you have arthritis. These are known as "knobbers."

A knobber is a hand-held device that has a "grip end," so it fits comfortably in your hand, and a projection (knob) that has a blunt, rounded end to press over the Pressure Point.

Knobbers come in different configurations and are made of various materials. I've used knobbers with small wood balls on the end and also knobbers made of a molded resin. They work great to penetrate the Pressure Point while relieving stress and pressure on your hands, wrists and arms.

If you use a knobber, find the Pressure Point with your hand first. Then use the knobber to treat the point.

As a word of caution, you can increase the amount of pressure exponentially using a hand knobber, bringing a person down to his knees! So be sure to go light and gradually increase pressure!

CHAPTER 11: NUTRITION

Nutrition plays an important role in your health. There is much written about nutrition and I wanted to share a few facts with you.

Pressure Points can form because of nutritional deficiencies. That's right—you can tighten up because of a lack of specific vitamins. I'll go over a few important ones.

Magnesium

Magnesium is a mineral which many feel is more important to supplement than calcium. It is needed to help the muscles relax. There are over 325 enzymatic reactions in the body that are magnesium-dependent. Magnesium is low in diabetics, those who work out a lot, children, senior citizens, people with heart problems, and more. My favorite form of magnesium supplement is one where you take a teaspoon of a powder, mix it in cold water and drink down. Oh, magnesium helps you relax and sleep well at night too!

Omega 3 Fatty Acids

Omega 3's are essential fatty acids that our bodies need but do not make. Many other animals, especially sea life, make their own Omega 3's. But we are dependent on getting them from outside sources.

When I mention "essential," this means it is needed for life and function.

The main effect of a lack of Omega 3's is inflammation. Inflammation IS the root of all evil, when it comes to pain and dysfunction in the body. Many researchers chuckle with all of the hype about cholesterol, knowing that it is inflammation that causes heart disease, not the former.

Omega 3's affect a certain kind of hormone that takes out inflammation in the body.

If you have pain, especially joint or back pain, you are probably lacking Omega 3's in your body. I recommend krill oil for Omega 3's. Krill oil has 300% greater Omega 3's than fish oil and is very absorbable. Along with Pressure Point Therapy, you'll find yourself doing much better with taking

Omega 3 fatty acids daily.

Vitamin D

When I was taking a course on nutrition many years ago, we were instructed not to prescribe Vitamin D. Why? Because it was in fortified milk. (Plus the body made its own "D" when out in the sun.) For years one would never hear about Vitamin D.

Today it is all over the Internet and newscasts. Vitamin D is one of the most researched substances.

This is what happened: it seemed that everything was going along A-OK until the early 1990's, when Vitamin D levels in society plunged. And they have been at the bottom ever since.

A number of events occurred in the early 1990's that brought on these changes: the Internet was launched; video games started becoming main-stream, and cable TV emerged with hundreds of channels.

In other words, we went inside and have stayed there ever since. Our Vitamin D factory has been shut down. It takes a good twenty minutes of sunlight on the bare skin to make Vitamin D.

When I say "bare," that means no sunscreen or blockers. An SPF 8, the lowest sunscreen one can purchase, blocks out over 90% of the good UV rays the body needs to make Vitamin D.

Ok, that's a bit of the background. Now the problems.

Low Vitamin D3 is linked to many conditions.

First is PAIN. Pain anywhere or everywhere in the body is associated with low Vitamin D levels in the blood.

Next is metabolic problems, like being overweight and having diabetes.

Then there are many hormone issues brought on by a lack of Vitamin D.

In fact, depending on the source, there are upwards of two thousand genes in the body that are dependant upon having Vitamin D present to work. So many things can get messed up.

The point is it is important to test the Vitamin D levels in your blood and then supplement to get your levels up. And keep them up. You will feel noticeably better.

More to Learn

Nutrition is a fascinating subject. If you're interested in reading more visit my Facebook page or my web site. I have many articles I write about vitamins, diet, nutrition and what not to do! My sites are

facebook.com/drpinkus

drpinkus.com

CHAPTER 12: TAKING CARE OF YOUR BODY

The body is an amazing creation. It can be fairly low-maintenance and will take care of itself if it is not abused too badly. The body is tough and can take a lot of stress.

Your body also has an innate mechanism to heal itself. Have you ever cut yourself only to find weeks later that the cut has completely vanished, not even leaving a scar? Your body healed itself.

If you have had your share of health problems or have been stuck on the "Medical Merry-Go-Round," then you will greatly benefit from Pressure Point Therapy. The key is, learn the technique and use it. Don't be discouraged that it "didn't work" after doing it a few times. This technique is amazing. The more you use it the more effective it seems to be. I even have my two dogs, Max and Miles, into it. They have been treated since being puppies. They love receiving Pressure Point Therapy. Plus, they are extremely healthy and need very little veterinary care.

Pressure Point Therapy is, in fact, a missing piece of health technology that I am now re-introducing. Writing this book is part of my efforts to help you, your family and community.

You now have the tools and soon, with practice, the know-how. Use Pressure Point Therapy to help others and yourself. You are now part of the Healing Arts.

Get to work.

We have a planet to heal!

Dr. Michael Pinkus

PART II: THE PRESSURE POINT TREATMENT CHARTS

THE PRESSURE POINT THERAPY TREATMENT CHARTS

Unlike acupressure or other similar therapies, Pressure Point Therapy is very easy to learn. Here you will find the Pressure Point Therapy Treatment Charts that you can follow to treat a variety of conditions.

The charts have been arranged in a "recipe" format so you can easily select a condition and have a corresponding chart to follow. Don't become too concerned about being precise. We are not too concerned with the accuracy of the points in relation to the chart. If a person has active Pressure Points, the charts will give you the proximity of where to find them. The rest is up to you to actually locate them on your recipient.

We place our emphasis on treating the Pressure Points so they release. We are also concerned with the recipient's well-being. He should have a good experience, knowing that something has changed for the better because of the treatment.

Many of the healing arts have lost the *healing* part. Most medical procedures are simply mechanical, and a person is treated as if they are having something done to a piece of meat! Add to this the abuses in over-prescribing drugs, unnecessary surgeries, and skyrocketing health care costs, and you have the current system of health care in this country.

Pressure Point Therapy works partly due to the science/technology behind it and greatly due to the fact that we emphasize communication between two people. It is personable. This is the "X-quality" that can never be reproduced with laboratory rats or in a test tube. To the degree that this intention is present, the technique will work wonderfully, even if the application is somewhat sloppy.

So, we encourage you to keep your attention on the person you are treating, rather than on the exactness of where the point is.

These charts represent the "Pressure Point Highways" in the body—where the majority of Pressure Points are located. As you become more familiar with the technique, you may find some points that are not listed on the charts. This is especially true because there are literally thousands of Pressure Points in the body. Nevertheless, the treatment is the same: when you find a tender Pressure Point treat it until it has released. You and your recipient will see the changes as you go.

The charts are laid out so all you have to do is follow the steps as numbered. Look over the chart before you treat your recipient. Have the charts literally next to you so you can reference the points as you are treating.

Many thanks will be coming your way for what you are doing with Pressure Point Therapy. I certainly thank you for being an active participant in helping make this a better and healthier world.

GENERAL PRESSURE POINTS FOR GREATER ENERGY AND VITALITY

Instructions: The steps below correspond with the chart on the opposite page.

Overview: Begin at the base of the skull/top of the neck and work each point going down. You can treat both left and right sides together. Return to the individual sore points and repeat the treatment on these areas.

1. Landmarks: Find the boney masses at the back of the head. They are located at the back of the skull, one on the left and one on the right, towards the outside. These "bumps" are part of your normal anatomy, so don't be concerned.

2. Starting Points: You'll start just below these masses. Slide your fingers down off of the bumps. You are now on the top of the spine. Put your thumbs together until they are touching and spread them out so they are about 1" on either side of the center of the spine. Press in and hold the area for about ten seconds.

3. Now make your way down the neck, into the back. Move downward about 1" to go the next points. As you work close to the actual spine, you will feel a series of bumps in the middle of the spine. Make sure you are about 1" to either side of these landmarks. Press and hold each point, both to the left and right of the center. Be sure to press in as your recipient exhales.

4. Note any tender points you encounter. After you have gone through the chart at least once, go back and treat those points individually again, one at a time.

5. You can repeat this pattern two to three times in one treatment.

Dr. P's Notes:

A. This is a great chart to help any person who needs to relax, who has been ill or recovering from an illness or who wants to "recharge" himself and become energized.

B. The recipient's body position can be either lying face down or sitting in a chair.

C. If you do this on your spouse, significant other, family member or friend before going to bed, the person will sleep much better. Try doing an exchange with someone so you both feel good!

D. This chart will also lower blood pressure, increase one's immune response, help blood flow and much more. So it is great for children, people under stress and seniors as well.

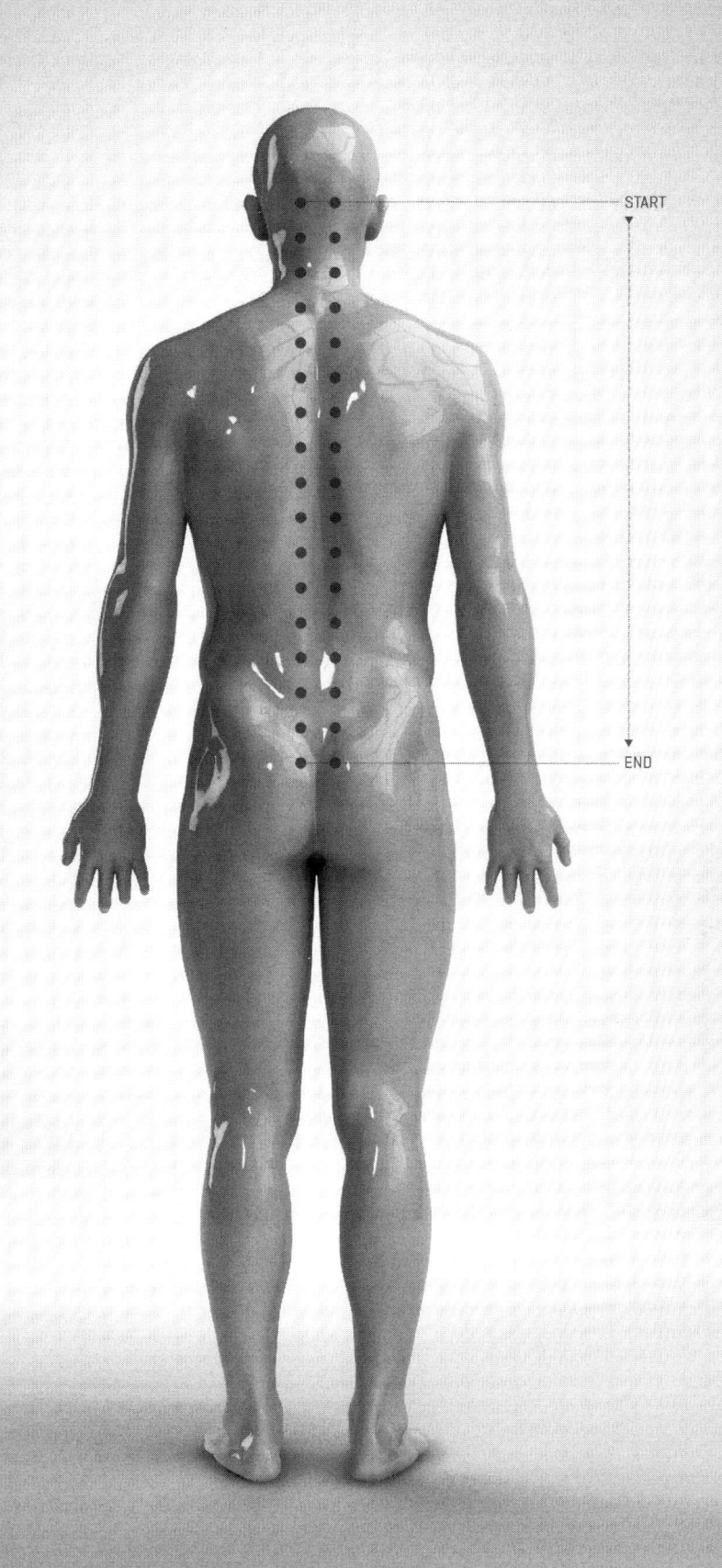

GENERAL PRESSURE POINTS FOR GREATER ENERGY AND VITALITY

LOW-BACK, SCIATIC AND HIP PAIN PRESSURE POINTS

Instructions: The steps below correspond with the numbers on the chart.

Overview: This chart will be used quite often as most people experience low-back pain in their lifetime at least once. It is very effective!

1. Low-back pain (or hip/sciatic pain) can be concentrated on one side or the other. It can also be diffuse, meaning all over. These Pressure Points are located 1" to either side of the spine. Do both sides, but one side at a time. Then concentrate on the side of the pain.

2. The gluteus Pressure Points are toward the side of the derriere where there is a "dimple." The points are deep within the muscle. Press down and inward at the same time. Watch the recipient's pain indicators as these can be very tender Pressure Points. You may have to repeat these points several times to get them to release.

3. The Pressure Points on the thighs are in the center. Treating one at a time, feel around until you find the tender spot. Use moderate pressure, not too hard here.

4. The Pressure Points below the knee are toward the outside of the calf, about 1" below the crease of the knee. They are normally very tender and are main points for low-back pain. Treat only one side at a time. Then continue down the calf with the other points.

5. Gently pinch the tissues between the Achilles' tendon. Hold for five to ten seconds.

Dr. P's Notes

A. You will most likely find one to three very tender, sometimes large, Pressure Points in the lower back area as in Step 1 above. These are the "traditional" areas that most practitioners who treat low-back pain work over and over again. You will give your recipient relief by treating these Pressure Points. But do it in small steps, not trying to handle each point in just one pass.

B. The Pressure Points over the gluteus area in Step 2 above are MAJOR Pressure Points. These are mostly ignored by practitioners. They tend to be deep. Sometimes you'll need to press directly inward to reach them. The sciatic nerve, the largest nerve in the body, goes through this area. So hip pain, leg pain, knee, ankle and even foot problems can be relieved by these points.

C. The thigh Pressure Points, as in Step 3 above, are completely missing in most treatment programs. They are usually tender and can give great relief to low-back pain. You'll want to press in the middle of the muscle and feel around until you "hit" the Pressure Point. You'll know when you did!

D. The Pressure Point just under the knee is the ONE! It is the most important point for low-back pain, and yet it is completely missed in most modern treatments for back pain. You'll find the point is EXTREMELY sore on most people, so take baby steps in handling the area. But it is the "Eureka" point for breaking the low-back pain pattern. Don't over-treat it. One or two passes only. Then find it again in subsequent Pressure Point treatments.

LOW-BACK, SCIATIC AND HIP PAIN PRESSURE POINTS

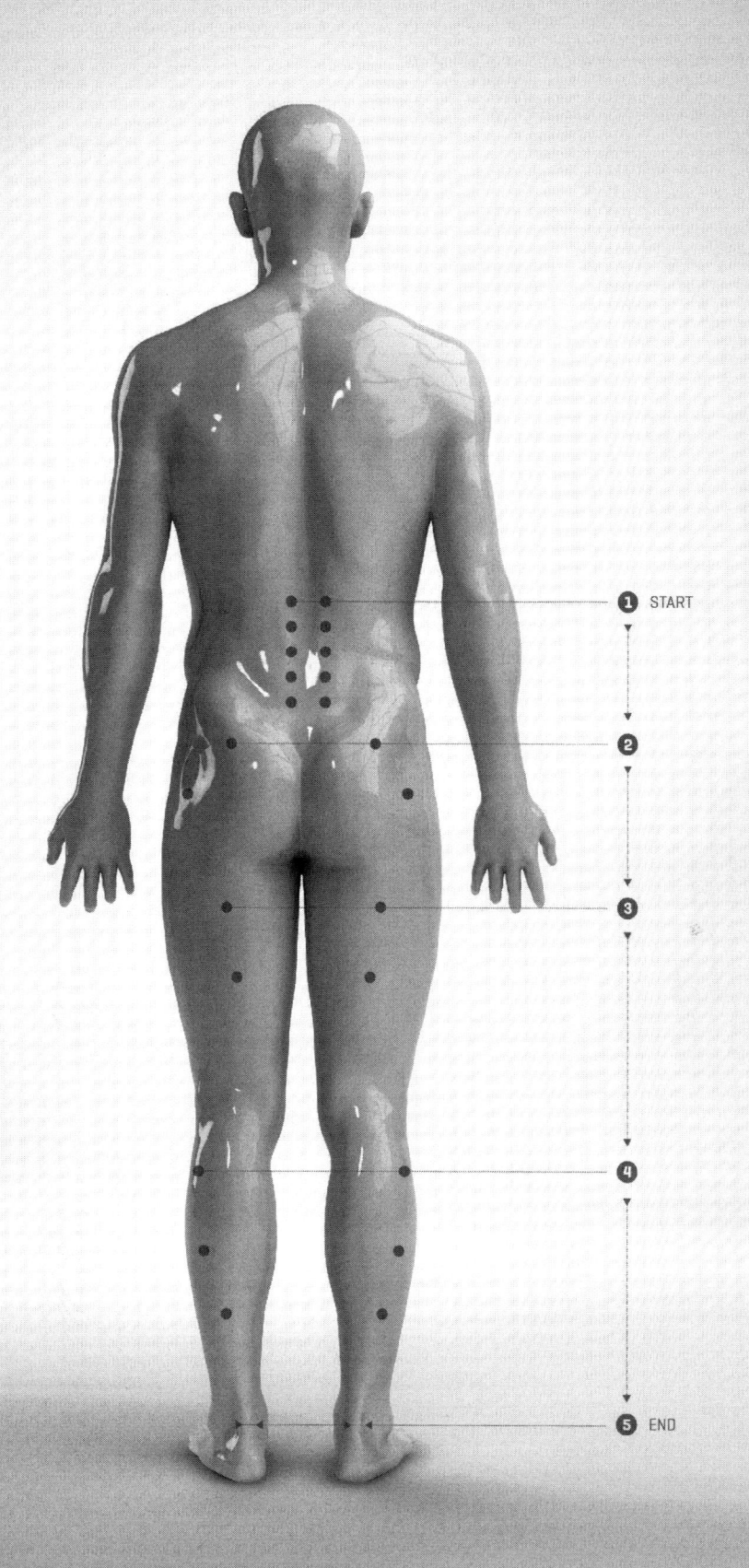

1. START
2.
3.
4.
5. END

LOW ENERGY PRESSURE POINTS

Instructions: The steps below correspond with the numbers on the charts.

Overview: The Low Energy Pressure Point Charts are divided into four sectional charts. Start with the first chart and continue through the remainder of the charts.

1. Treat points 1" to either side of the spine. Do both sides together. Repeat on painful Pressure Points, treating only one at a time.

2. Treat the points at the top of the shoulders, starting closest to the neck and moving outward. Repeat on painful points.

3. Gently treat the points on the center of the chest. Start at that top of the chest and work your way down. The last point is in the center of the chest.

4. Treat these two points last. They are located 1" below the center-point of the collarbone. These points are often tender.

Dr. P Notes:

A. If you're feeling tired, run-down or low-energy, these charts work great! They can be done at home, work or even on a plane.

B. Many of the Low Energy Pressure Points can be done by yourself. Charts 3 and 4 are easy to do anywhere and are very effective for a "pick-me-up!"

C. If working with a chronic low energy condition, such as mono, chronic fatigue syndrome, exhaustion, etc., do the points on these charts daily. Your recipient will notice an improvement in his energy.

D. When working the points on or near the chest, please be mindful when working with a female recipient.

E. The points on Chart 4 can be very painful. Work slowly. These are very powerful Pressure Points in terms of opening up the energy flow in the body.

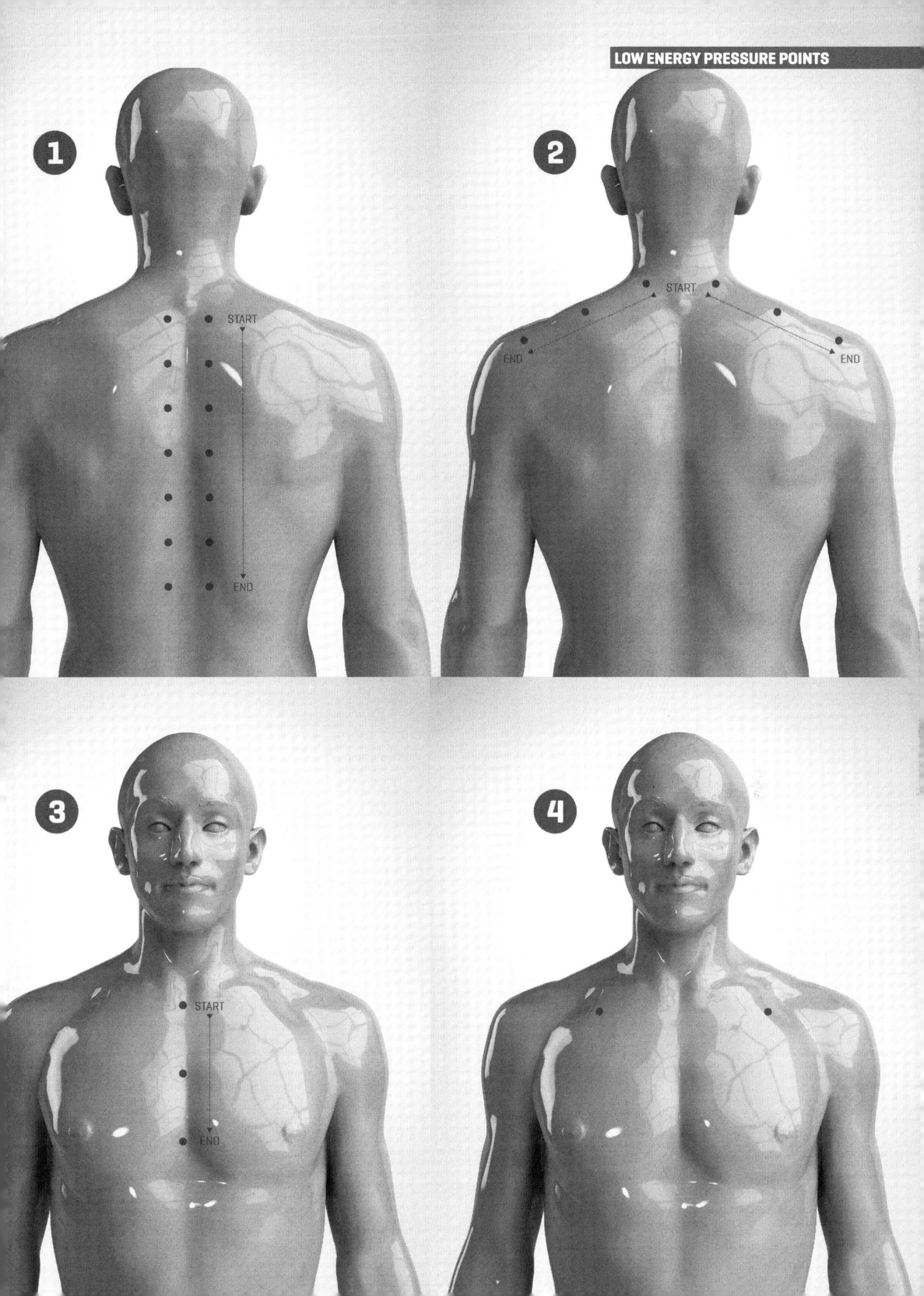

LOW ENERGY PRESSURE POINTS

NECK PAIN PRESSURE POINTS

Instructions: The steps below correspond with the numbers on the charts.

Overview: Refer to the chart on the left for Step 1 below and chart on the right for Steps 2 and 3.

1. Neck pain is usually found mostly on one side. Begin on the side of pain. Because neck pain is often related to Pressure Points in the upper back (as well as the neck), begin in the neck and work your way down into the upper back. Do one side then the other. Repeat on sore points.

2. These points are on the base of the skull, below the boney masses at the back of the head. Many of the neck muscles insert at these points, so they may be tender. Treat a bit at a time and repeat until the tenderness lightens.

3. Treat the top-of-the-shoulder points last. These are almost always sore.

Dr. P Notes:

A. Many of the neck muscles start in the upper- and mid-back area. A person, like someone with a "stiff neck" or even a full-blown whiplash, will feel his neck hurting, whereas the actual Pressure Points causing the pain are in the upper or mid back. This is why Step 1 above is important. You will always find Pressure Points in the upper and mid back associated with neck pain.

B. The points at the back of the head, as discussed in Step 2 above, are points where several neck muscles attach. These can be very sore, so be light! Treat these areas several times, if need be, so the tenderness lessens. These are also points that can involved in headaches. See chart "Headache and Jaw Pain (TMJ) Pressure Points."

C. The top of the shoulder will have "good ones" too—almost always. When these are successfully treated the recipient will often state something like, "The bricks are off my shoulders!"

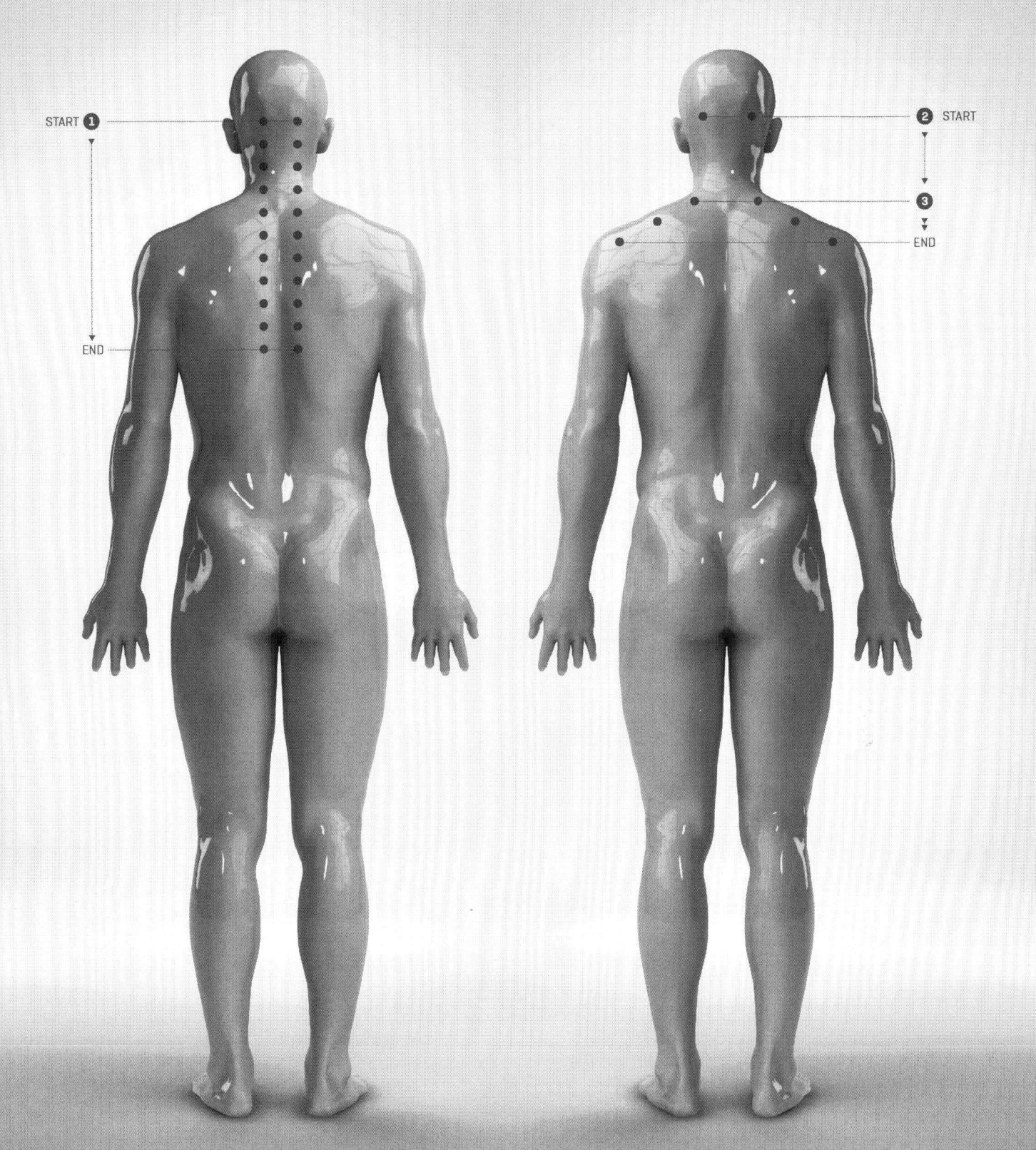

NECK PAIN PRESSURE POINTS

UPPER- OR MID-BACK PAIN, PAIN-BETWEEN-THE-SHOULDERS PRESSURE POINTS

Instructions: The steps below correspond with the numbers on the charts.

Overview: Refer to the chart on the left for Step 1 below and the chart on the right for Steps 2 and 3.

1. Start with the points in the neck and work your way down through the mid back. Do both sides together. Work over the tender Pressure Points. You may find sore points especially in the vicinity of the shoulder blades.

2. Next treat the areas in the upper shoulder area. Repeat treatment on tender Pressure Points found.

3. Work the areas on the inside of the shoulder blades last. Spend extra time on the painful Pressure Points.

Dr. P Notes:

A. The Pressure Points in the neck are associated with the upper- and mid-back muscles, so that's why we start in this region.

B. Pain between the shoulders and mid-back pain are often times related to spasms between the ribs. The Pressure Points going down the back, as in Step 1, and also along the inside of the shoulder blades, as in Step 3, are often times related to these rib muscle spasms. They will be very tender, so do multiple lighter treatments on the very sore points.

C. Using the breathing techniques described in Part 1 of this book will help release these areas. Instruct your recipient to breathe out when you push down over the point. Also, these charts provide great relief for those suffering from this sort of pain. They will in turn, be able to take a deeper breath without effort!

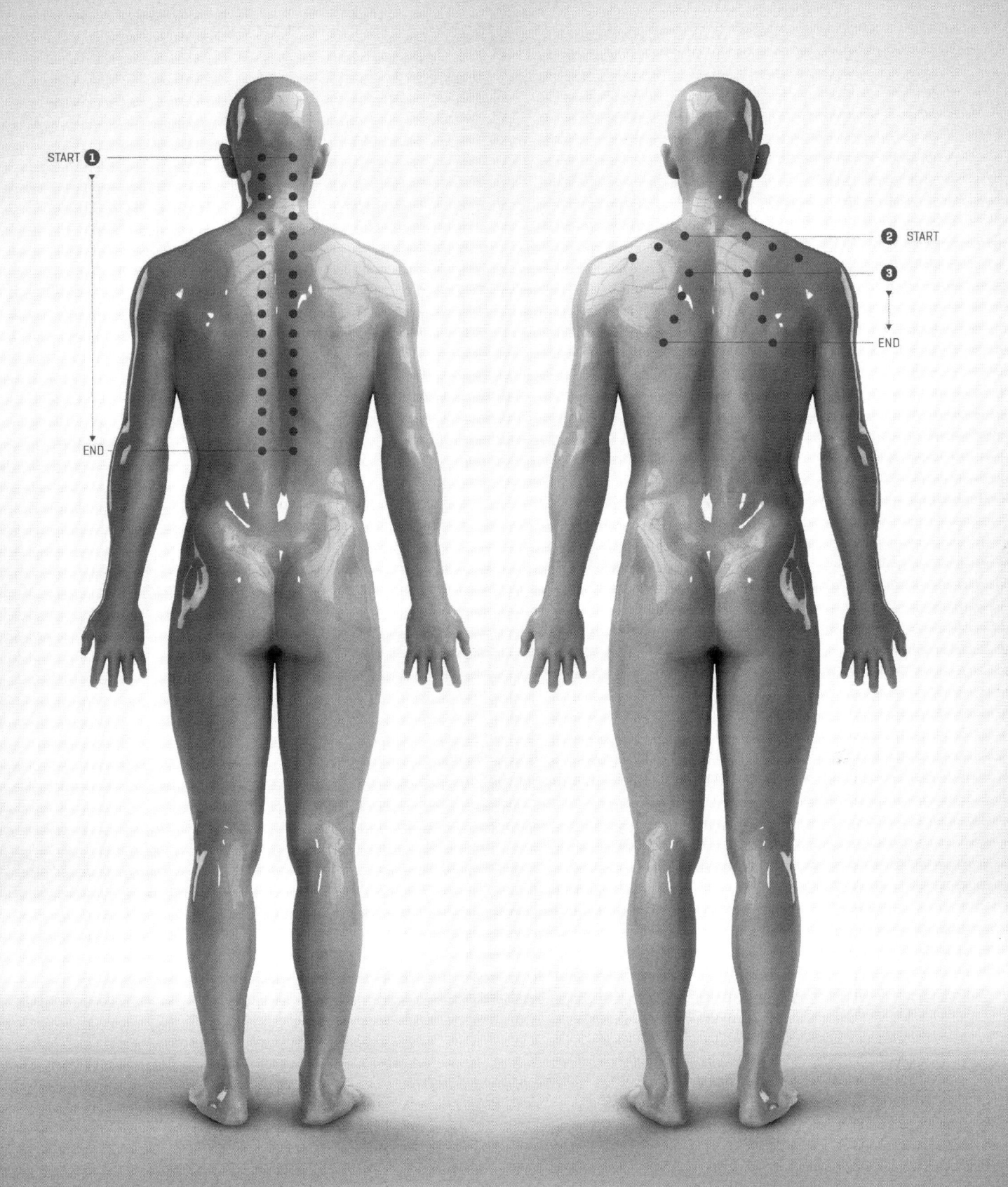

UPPER- OR MID-BACK PAIN, PAIN-BETWEEN-THE-SHOULDERS PRESSURE POINTS

PRESSURE POINTS FOR LUNG PROBLEMS

Instructions: The steps below correspond with the numbers on the charts.

Overview: Refer to the chart on the left for Step 1 and the chart on the right for Steps 2 and 3.

1. Starting in the neck, treat the Pressure Points on both sides of the spine and work your way down to the mid back. Do both sides together and repeat on the tender points.

2. Beginning at the ball of the shoulder, work your way down the arm. Finish by "pinching" the web of the hand. Do one side at a time. Repeat on tender Pressure Points.

3. Treat the Pressure Points in the mid-chest area. You can treat these one side at a time or together. They may be quite sore. Repeat on tender Pressure Points.

4. Treat these Pressure Points last. They are located 1" below the center of the collarbone. Treat one at a time. Will often be tender so treat a bit at a time and repeat.

Dr. P Notes:

A. The nerves in the neck travel into the lungs. This is why we start in this area.

B. The Pressure Points in the mid back will often be very tight, especially if one has been coughing or if one has asthma. Often, breathing will improve when the mid-back Pressure Points have been gone over.

C. The Pressure Points going down the arm are associated with the lungs. You'll find tender spots working your way down the arms. This is true especially with smokers!

D. The mid-chest points also can be very sore. Watch your recipient's indicators: if he is squirming or grimacing, lighten your touch! Be mindful of this area when working with females to avoid contacting the breast area.

E. The Pressure Point under the collarbone is a major lung point. You may have to feel around to find it. But it is always sore on one side or the other (or both sides). Treated correctly, it almost always gives great relief to lung sufferers.

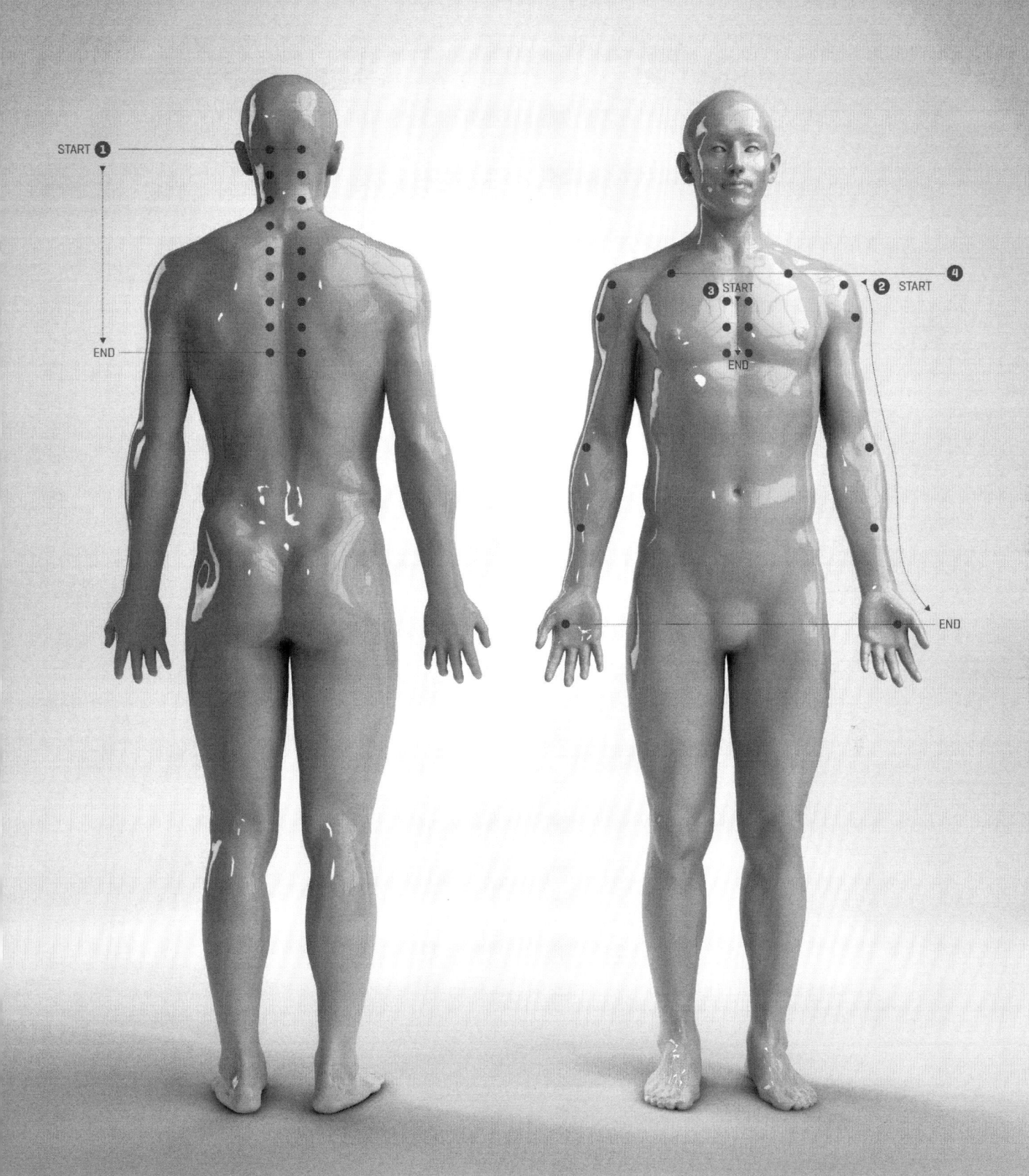

PRESSURE POINTS FOR LUNG PROBLEMS

PRESSURE POINTS FOR HAND, WRIST AND ELBOW PAIN

Instructions: The steps below correspond with the numbers on the charts.

Overview: Steps 1 and 2 correspond to the chart on the left. For Step 3 reference the chart on the right.

1. Treat only the side of the body one is experiencing pain on. Start in the neck and work your way down over the top of the shoulder. Note any tender points and then repeat.

2. Treat the points in the triceps area. These are often very tender so treat lightly and repeat until pain is lessened. Continue working your way down through the back of the forearm and into the hand. Repeat on tender points.

3. Treat the points on the front of the shoulder, working your way down the biceps, the front of the forearm and the hand. Repeat on tender points.

Dr. P Notes:

A. The Pressure Points in the neck are connected to the arm, wrist and hand. This is why we start in here.

B. Pain below the elbow is sometimes caused by Pressure Points on the top of the shoulders.

C. The points in the triceps and biceps are often very sore. Treat lightly and repeat to release them.

D. The Pressure Point just below the elbow is a "doozie." Again treat lightly and repeat.

E. You'll find incredible relief using these charts. With computers and even hand-held electronic devices, wrist and hand pain are very common. I've had great responses even with post-surgical cases who did not respond well to wrist or hand surgery!

PRESSURE POINTS FOR HAND, WRIST AND ELBOW PAIN

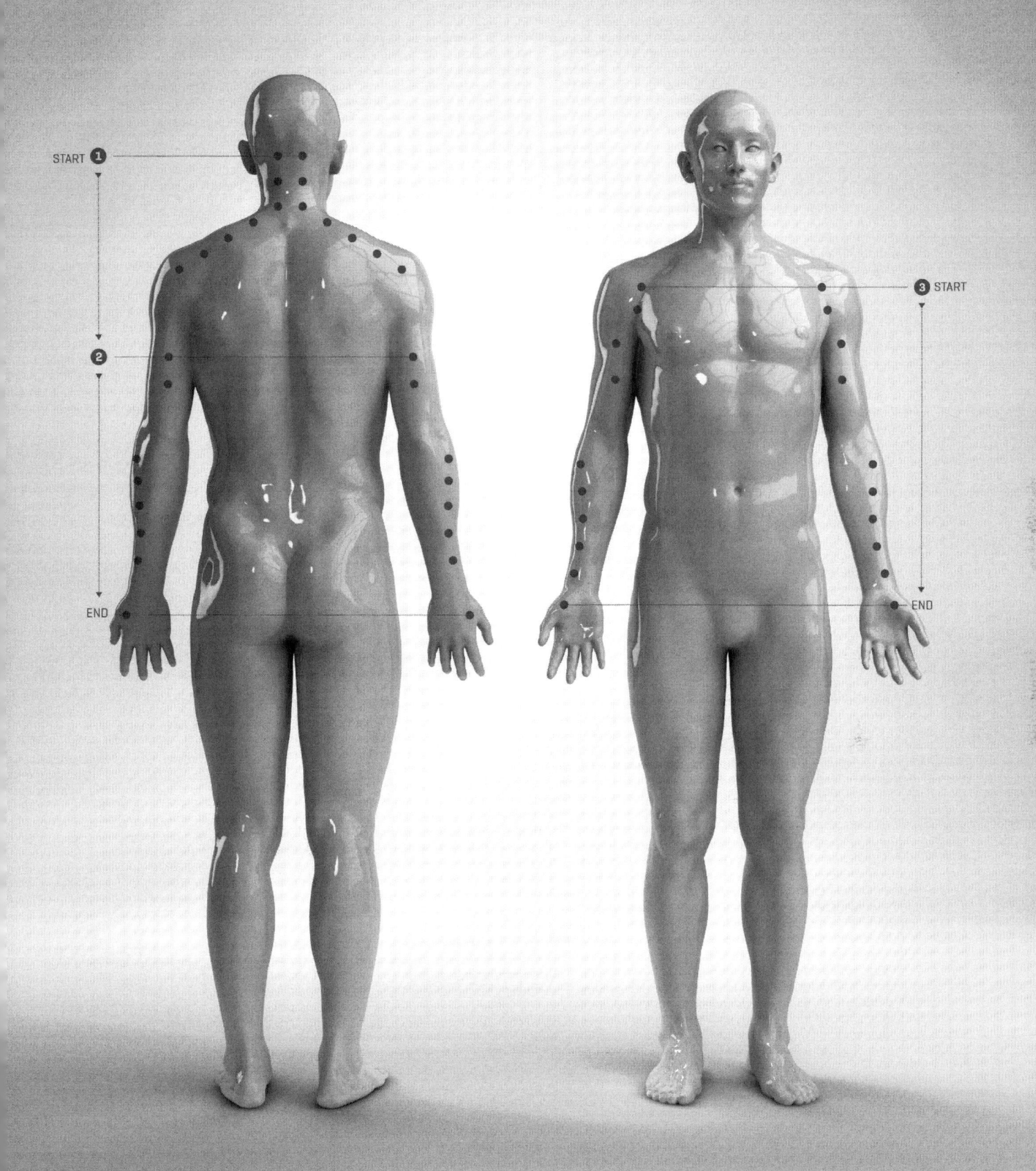

PRESSURE POINTS FOR SINUSES, ALLERGIES, HEAD COLDS AND CONGESTION

Instructions: The steps below correspond with the numbers on the charts.

Overview: This chart is great for any of these congestion-forming conditions! Follow Steps 1-3 below.

1. Begin by treating the Pressure Points directly above the eyebrows. These correspond to the upper sinuses. They are located on the forehead, just above the eyebrow. Treat one at a time. You may have to feel around a bit to find the tender spot. One or both may be tender. Repeat on the tender points.

2. Treat the Pressure Points on the face. These are located just to the side of the nose, in a small "valley." Treat one point at a time. They will be very tender when your recipient is congested. These points are associated maxillary sinuses: the main sinuses areas that are chronically congested in these cases. Repeat the treatment.

3. Treat the chest points. The points under the collarbone will often be quite tender so treat lightly and repeat. Then treat the points on the chest. Repeat on tender Pressure Points.

Dr. P Notes:

A. The Pressure Points above the eyes are great for sinus pressure and sinus headaches.

B. The points to the side of the nose, in Step 2 above are the major sinus Pressure Points. Be prepared to have your recipient's sinuses drain! So have tissues available.

C. You can alternate between the upper and lower sinus points. Again, these are very effective.

D. The points below the collarbone are associated with the "main drain" for the head and neck. When these Pressure Points are tightened up they can actually block the drainage of the head. Constant congestion and infections are the results. I've had numerous recipients report that their entire head and neck drained following the treatment of these areas.

E. The two points on the chest complete the treatment. They can be sore. Be mindful of this area if your recipient is female.

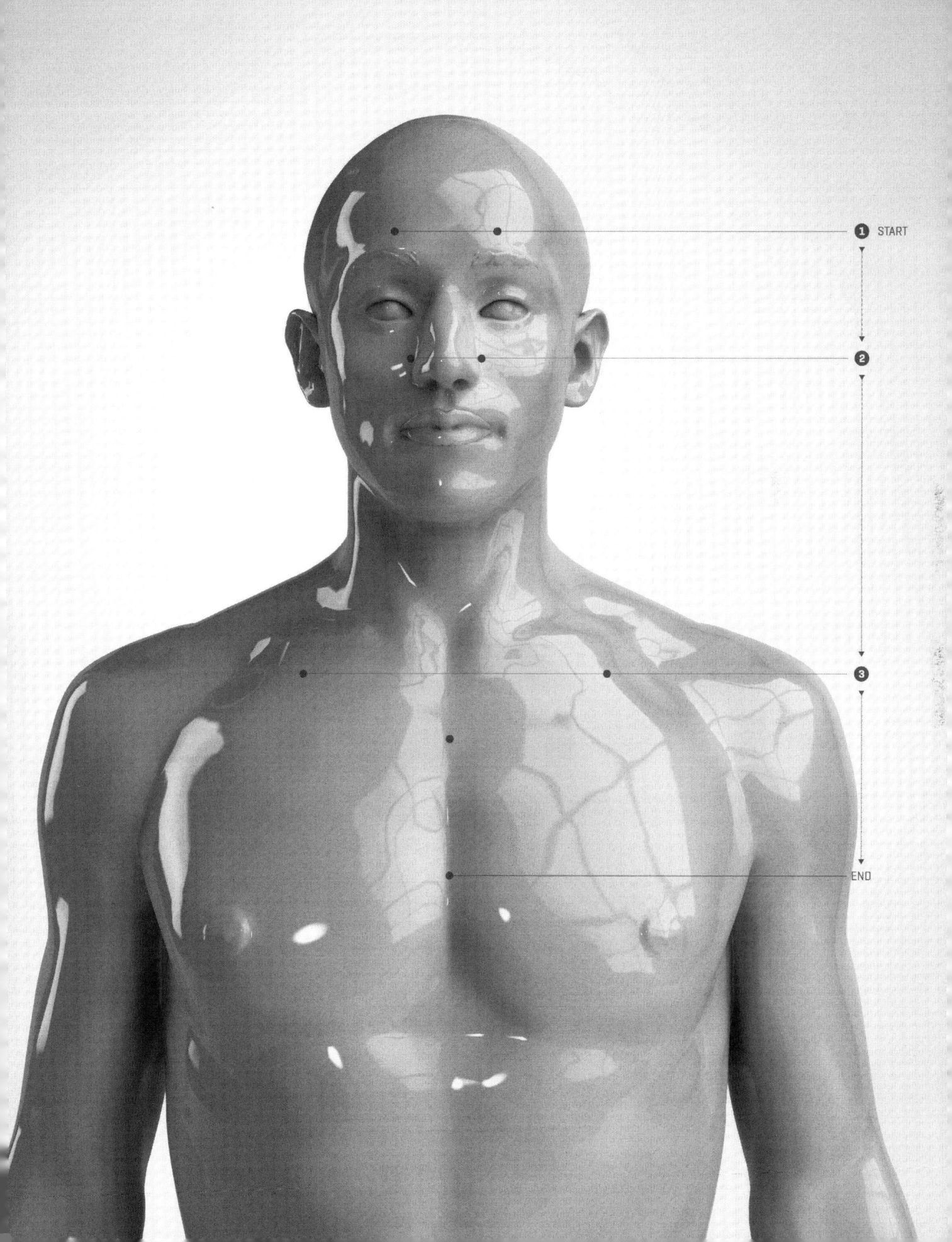

PRESSURE POINTS FOR SINUSES, ALLERGIES, HEAD COLDS AND CONGESTION

1 START

2

3

END

HEADACHE AND JAW PAIN (TMJ) PRESSURE POINTS

Instructions: The steps below correspond with the numbers on the charts.

Overview: The Headache and TMJ Pressure Points are found on three sectional charts. Follow Steps 1-6, in order.

1. Start with the Pressure Points at the upper back and work your way up into the neck. Note tender points and repeat. You can treat both sides together.

2. The Pressure Points at the base of the skull can be quite tender. Work gently until they are released.

3. Now work the points from the back of the head over the temple and into the jaw. Several of these Pressure Points will be very sore, so work gently on them and repeat.

4. The Pressure Point over the jaw is always very sore. Work it over with very light pressure until it releases, which may take several passes.

5. These points are also associated with the top sinuses. They are located just above the eyebrows. You may have to feel around to find them. Do one at a time and hold until it releases.

6. Treat these points last. When tight, they can hold in congestion in the head and neck.

Dr. P Notes:

A. There are several different types of headaches and these charts are effective with most. Your recipient will think you have "magic powers" in your hands when his headaches vanish after you have performed the Pressure Point Therapy treatment!

B. For migraine sufferers, treat often, especially when one does NOT have a headache! As a result, migraines will be shorter in duration and less frequent.

C. Many headaches, especially tension headaches, begin in the neck and upper back. This is why we start there. Your recipient will have no idea that these Pressure Points are active because the pain is in his forehead, not his neck or back!

D. The Pressure Points above the ear, over the temple and over the jaw are often VERY tender. So watch your recipient's indicators, use the breathing technique and lighten up so these points release. The headache goes away with these points, by the way!

E. Over-the-counter pain relievers and prescription drugs mask the pain and do nothing for the actual cause of headaches (i.e. Pressure Points). With constant use, drugs actually lock Pressure Points into spasm and perpetuate the condition.

HEADACHE AND JAW PAIN (TMJ) PRESSURE POINTS

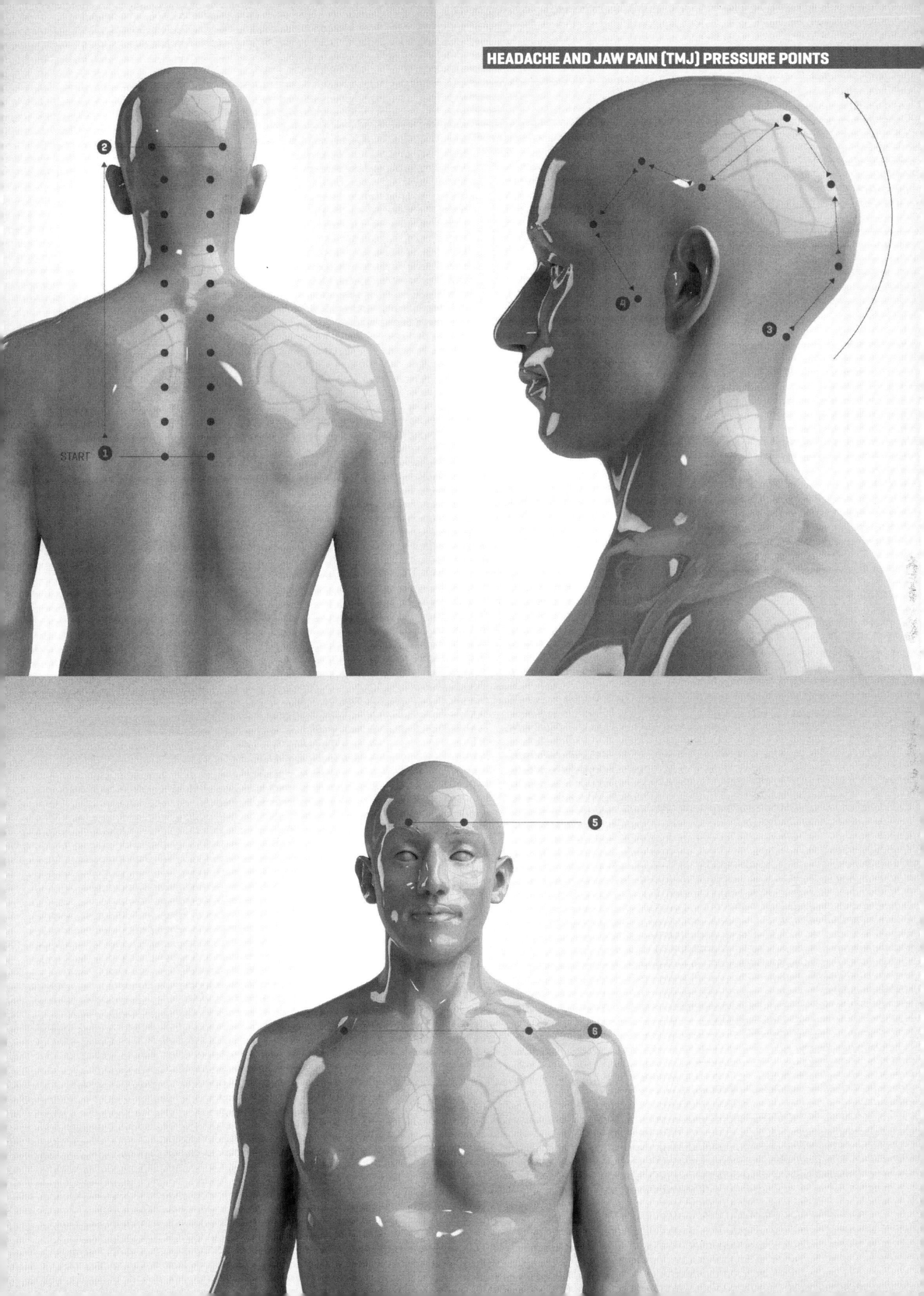

START

PRESSURE POINTS FOR HORMONAL CONDITIONS (PMS, ETC.)

Instructions: The steps below correspond with the numbers on the charts.

Overview: The Pressure Points for these conditions are found on two sectional charts: Steps 1-3 on the left chart and Steps 4-5 on the right chart. Step 6 has points located on both charts.

1. Treat the Pressure Points down the back both sides at the same time. Repeat on sore points.

2. Repeat the lower back Pressure Points several times. These may be very tender.

3. These Pressure Points are over the sacrum, a triangular-shaped bone at the base of the spine. The points are located specifically on the outer edge of this bone. Treat one side at a time and repeat on sore points.

4. The Pressure Points here are just behind the hip bone. They may be quite tender so work one point at a time and repeat if necessary.

5. The outside of the thigh contains these "hidden" Pressure Points. They are a must to help relieve these conditions. Be very gentle as they are very tender. Repeat two or three times and the point will greatly lighten up.

6. Treat the points on the feet and ankles last. These points often have a burning feeling when treated. Be gentle and repeat.

Dr. P Notes:

A. These charts can be used for a number of conditions having to do with the reproductive organs and system. They may be effective for menopausal symptoms and other female hormonal conditions.

B. Each step above gives great relief. Take your time and treat the sore Pressure Points until they release.

C. The points on the outside of the thigh are some of the most potentially painful ones in the body! But the results are instant and spectacular.

D. Repeat often. Most PMS and hormonal problems will slowly normalize by using these charts.

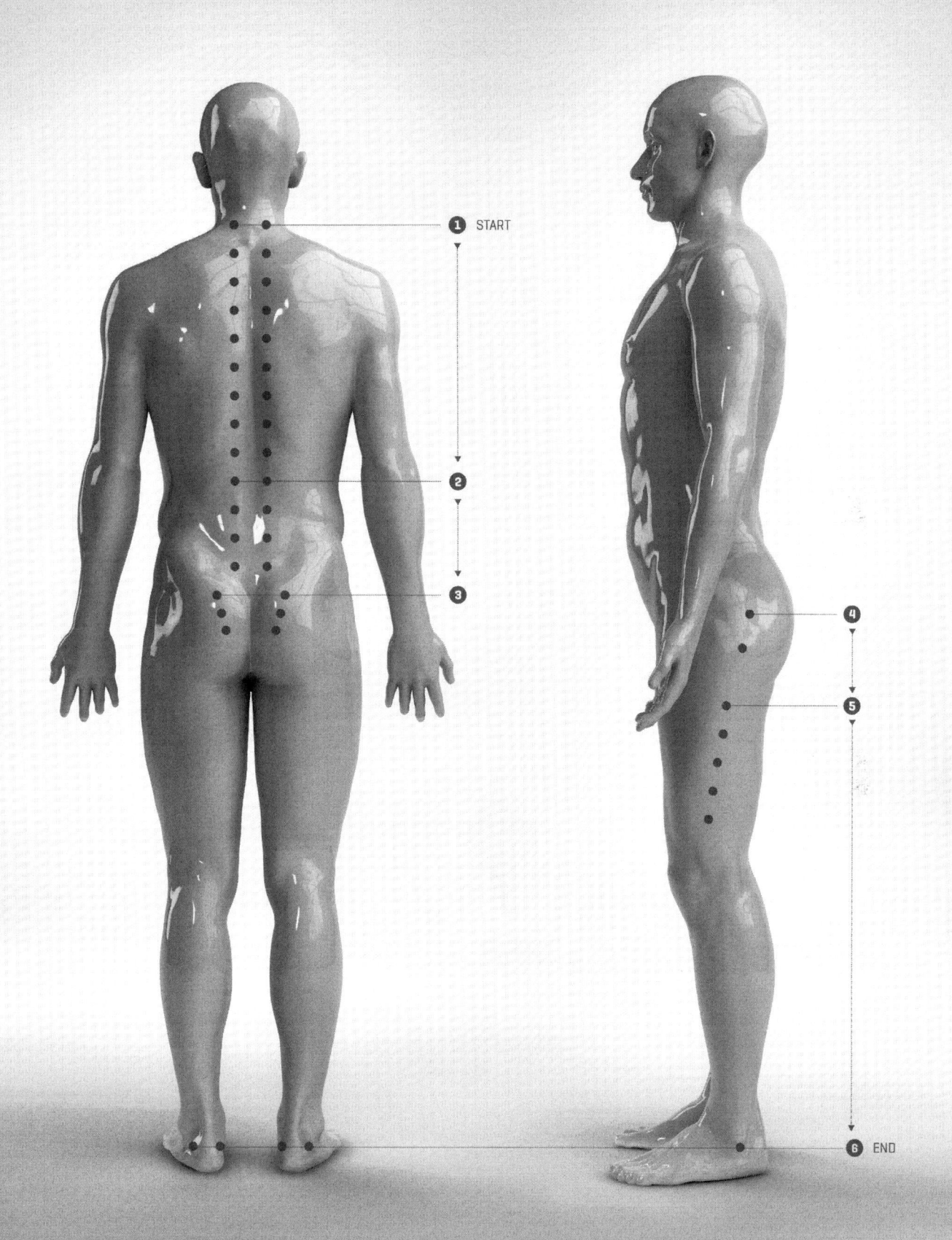

PRESSURE POINTS FOR HORMONAL CONDITIONS (PMS, ETC.)

1. START
2.
3.
4.
5.
6. END

PRESSURE POINTS FOR DIGESTIVE PROBLEMS

Instructions: The steps below correspond with the numbers on the charts.

Overview: The chart contains the Pressure Points for digestive problems. Work the chart frequently for best results.

1. Start with the Pressure Points just below the boney masses at the back of the skull. These may be tender so work in small steps and repeat until the points release.

2. The Pressure Points in the upper and mid back correspond to the stomach, intestines, pancreas, liver and gall bladder. You will find several tender Pressure Points here or one or two "big ones." Repeat on painful points until released.

3. The last points are in the web of the hand, between the thumb and forefinger. Pinch together and hold until Pressure Point releases. May be very tender and could take a little longer to release.

Dr. P Notes:

A. The Pressure Points at the top of the neck correspond with a major nerve which starts in the head, travels through the neck, lungs, heart, digestive tract and all the way down to the large intestine. When these neck Pressure Points are triggered, one could have dozens of symptoms, including numerous digestive tract disorders. Suffice it to say, the treatments of these Pressure Points are very effective!

B. The nervous system is "wired" in such a way that there are few sensory pain nerves in the digestive tract. The body therefore "externalizes" sensations, mostly to the upper- and mid-back areas. Step 2 above addresses the major "circuit breakers" related to the digestive tract. The relief a person will experience after a treatment is incredible.

C. Along with treating Pressure Points, diet and nutritional supplements (like probiotics and digestive enzymes) are obviously important from a holistic point of view in handling digestive problems.

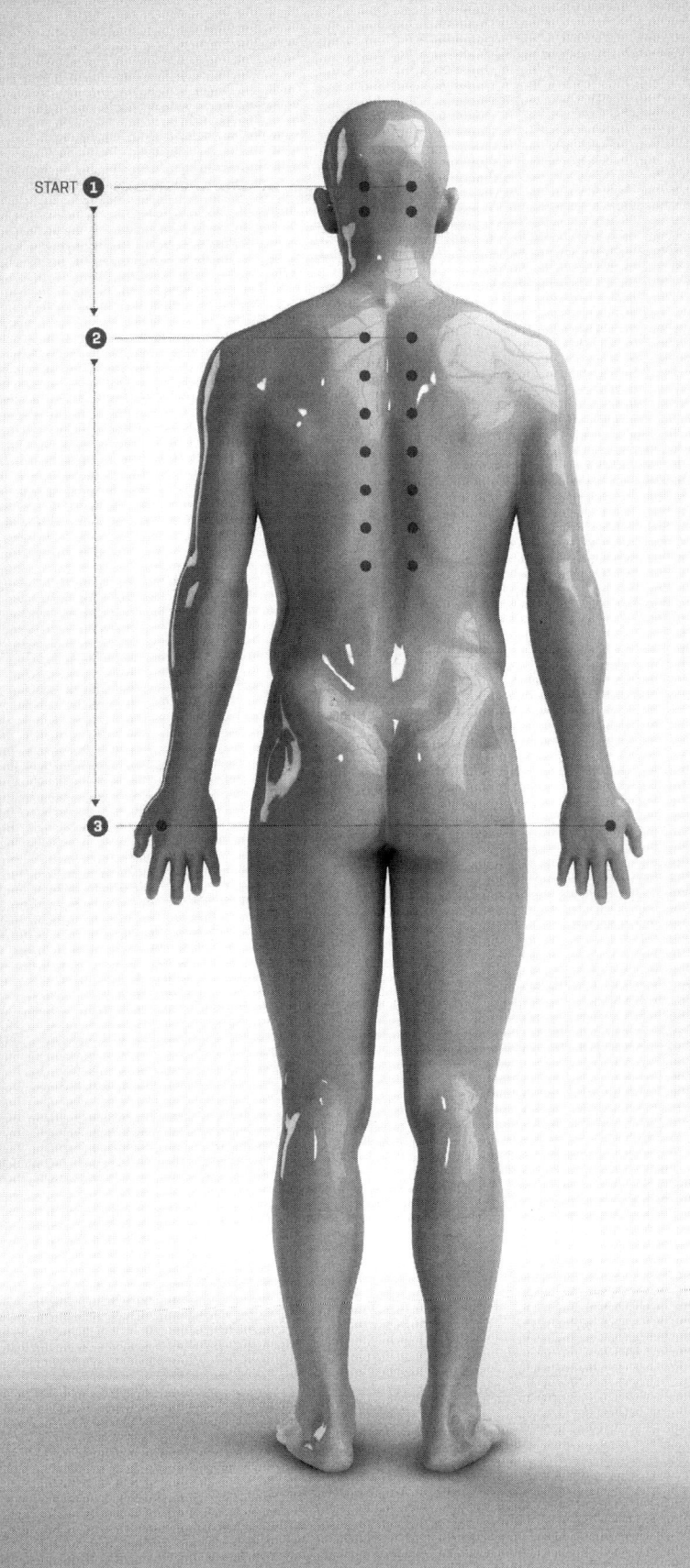

PRESSURE POINTS FOR DIGESTIVE PROBLEMS

PRESSURE POINT FOR SHOULDER PAIN

Instructions: The steps below correspond with the numbers on the charts.

Overview: Steps 1 and 2 correspond with the top sectional chart. Steps 3 and 4 with the side view chart. Step 5 goes with the front sectional chart. Note, charts only show right side but the points are same for the left side.

1. Begin by treating the Pressure Points on the inside of the shoulder blade. Do only one side at a time. Repeat on sore points.

2. Starting at the top of the shoulder work the Pressure Points traveling into the shoulder itself. The last three or four points can be very sore so be gentle and repeat on painful ones.

3. Work on the Pressure Points towards the back of the shoulder working your way down the arm, just above the elbow. The areas over the triceps muscle will also be very tender.

4. Treat the Pressure Points on the side of the shoulder.

5. Starting on the chest, in the groove between the chest and the shoulder, treat the Pressure Points on the front of the shoulder, going into the arm. Again, any of these can be real tender so do several passes if need be.

Dr. P Notes:

A. The shoulder is the only joint in the body that is held together by several muscles. If Pressure Points block the function of even one muscle, an imbalance occurs. Thus, doing Pressure Point Therapy on the shoulder gives great relief.

B. Many of the Pressure Points on these charts are deep in the tissue. So take your time to feel around. Be sure to apply as much pressure as your recipient can handle and then do several passes until the points release.

C. With chronic shoulder problems, do treatments often. You will see great results!

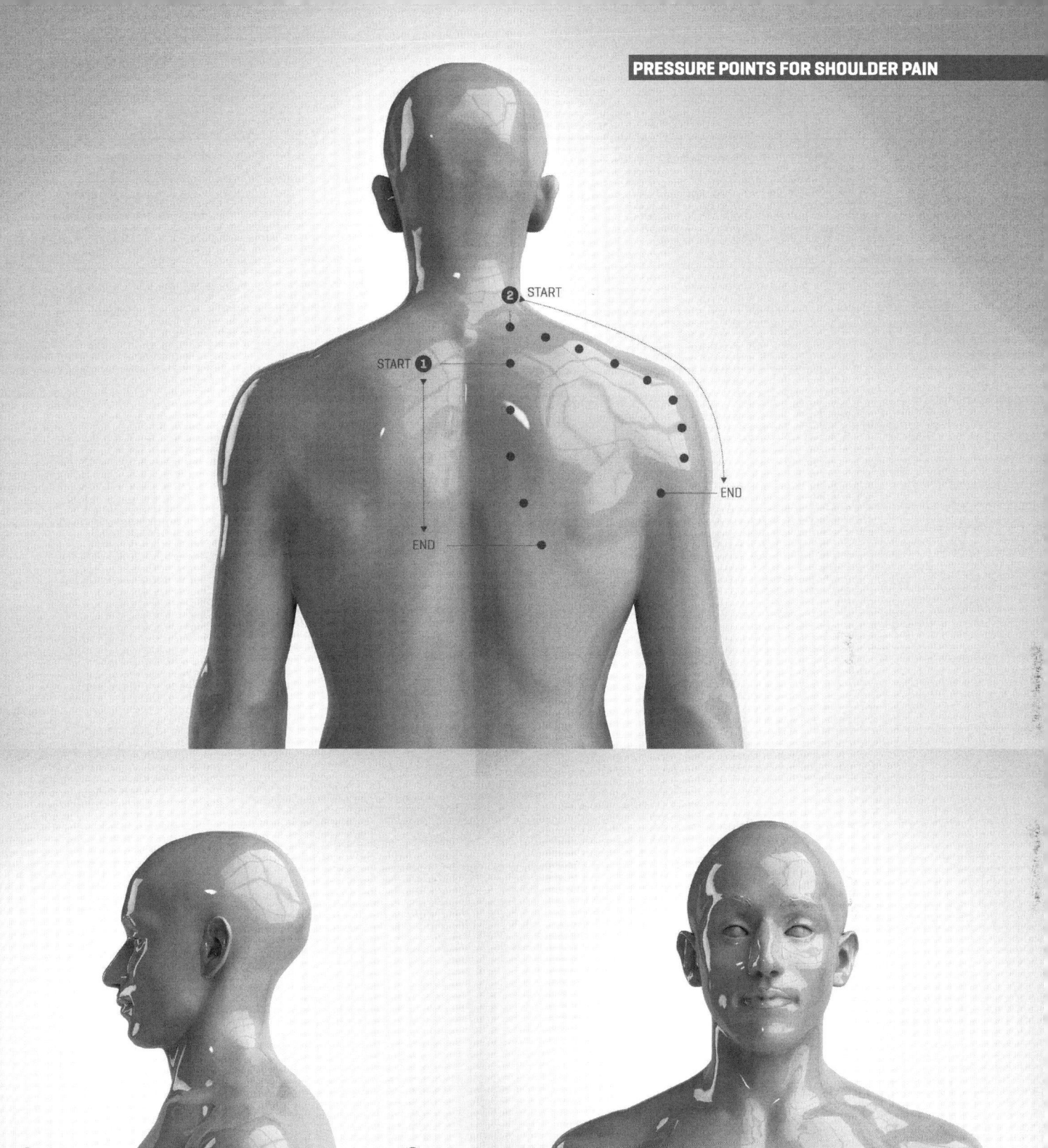

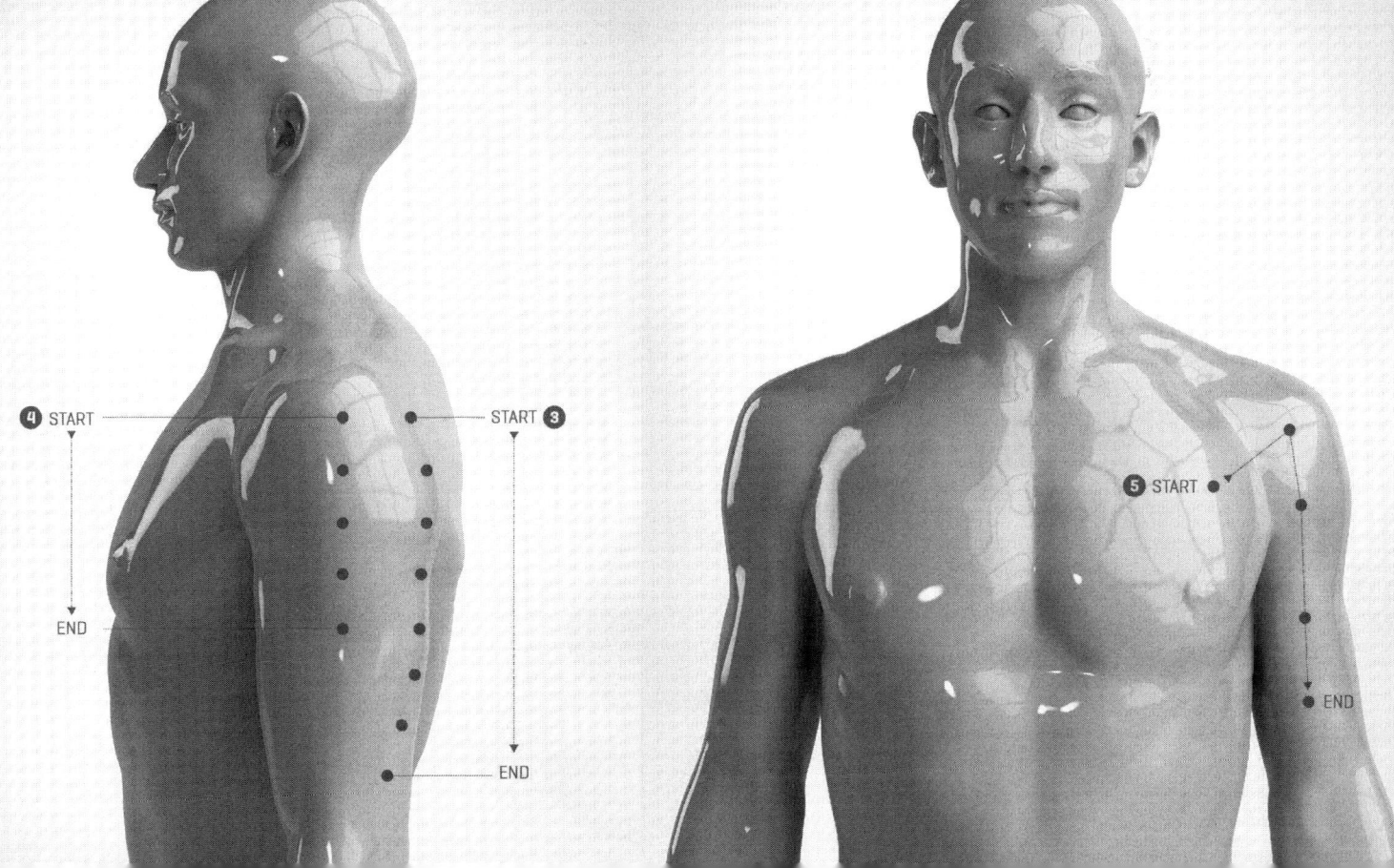

PRESSURE POINTS FOR SHOULDER PAIN

KNEE PAIN PRESSURE POINTS

Instructions: The steps below correspond with the numbers on the charts.

Overview: The top sectional chart is for Steps 1 and 2. The front chart for Steps 3 and 4. The side chart or Step 5. Note: Charts show points only on the right side but they are the same on the left side.

1. Begin with the lower back Pressure Points. The points on the side of knee pain may be more tender. Repeat on sore areas. Do both sides.

2. The Pressure Points in the gluteus area will be tender. Treat these and continue down the leg. In the thigh area the Pressure Points are in the middle, and below the knee they are located more to the outside of the calf.

3. Work the two points above and below the knee. These are always quite tender. Repeat until they release.

4. Continue down the front of the leg to the outside of the shin.

5. The points on the outside of the thigh will be very tender. Be gentle and do several passes until these release. Continue working the points below the knee as well.

Dr. P Notes:

A. Knee pain persists because practitioners fail to treat the Pressure Points in the lower back and hip areas. It is here where the nerves that end up in the knee originate. So expect great results in doing these charts.

B. Many times a person has arthritis or torn cartilages in the knees and will need surgical treatment (or already has had surgery). Pressure Point Therapy will still help. I worked on a US Olympic athlete who had had seven knee surgeries. After my treatments he won the Silver Medal for the team! (Do not treat a person who has just had surgery. Let them heal up for a few weeks then gently proceed.)

C. Any one of these Pressure Points will be extremely sore. So treat within the pain tolerance of your recipient and go over the areas once again. Do frequent treatments, especially if rehabbing the knee.

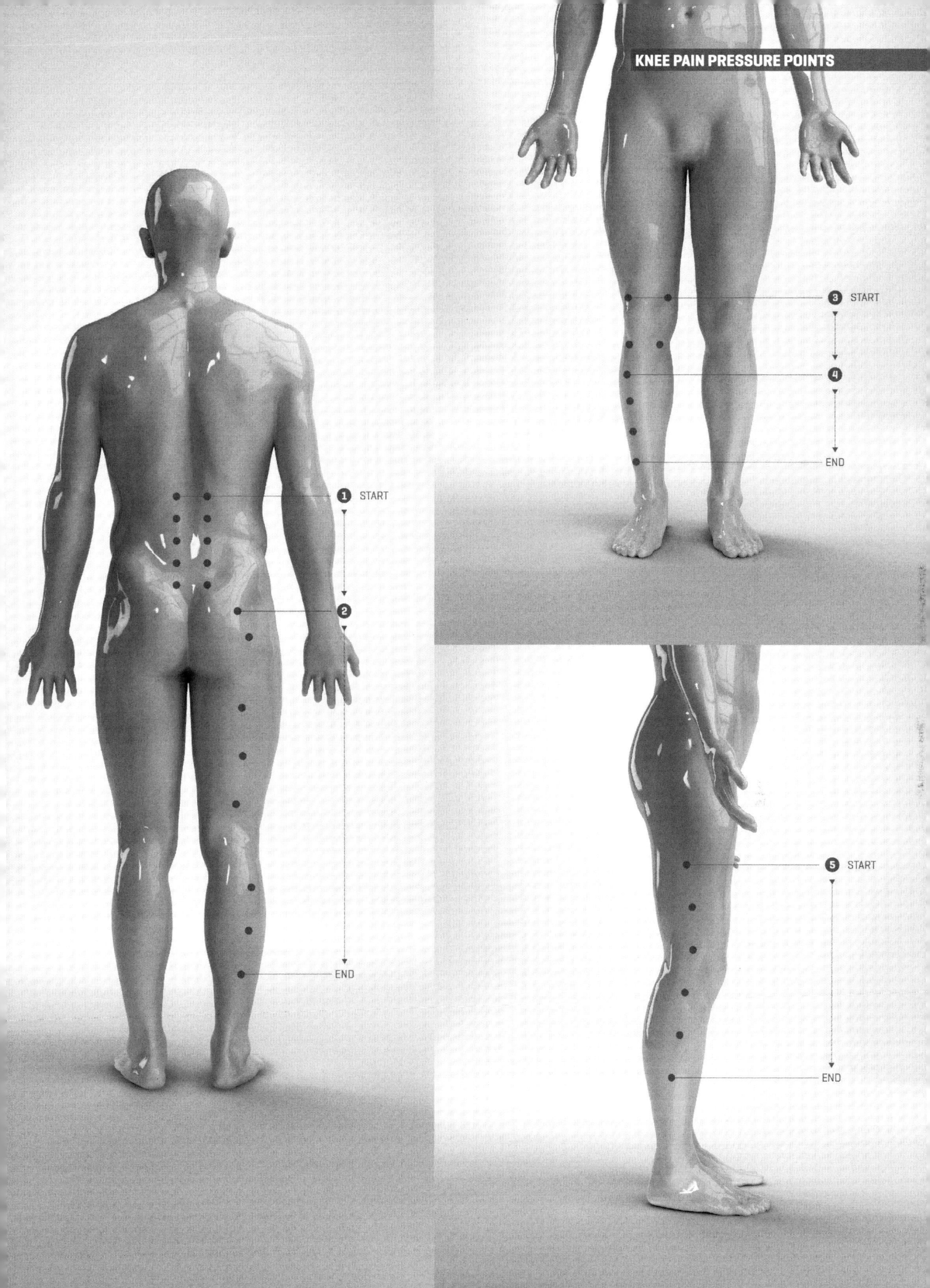

KNEE PAIN PRESSURE POINTS

PRESSURE POINTS FOR COLD AND FLU SYMPTOMS

Instructions: The steps below correspond with the numbers on the charts.

Overview: The sectional chart on the left is for Steps 1 and 2. The upper right chart for Step 3 and lower right chart for Steps 4 and 5.

1. Treat the Pressure Points in the neck and in the upper- and mid-back areas first. You can treat both sides together. Repeat on tender Pressure Points.

2. The lower back Pressure Points are useful for the flu, when one is aching or sore. Treat both together and repeat the painful points.

3. Next treat the two points on top of the shoulders. These are helpful for fevers and neck pain.

4. The Pressure Points on the face will open up congested sinuses. Treat these points repeatedly until the tenderness over the points lessens and/or sinus congestion opens up.

5. Find the Pressure Points 1" below the collarbone. Here you will find a very tender spot that, once opened, will drain the head and throat. Work on one side at a time.

Dr. P Notes:

A. These charts are very effective in helping a person recover from the cold or flu. The body, in response to viral or bacteria infection, aggravates Pressure Points. This results in pain, low energy and lower immune response. Treat these Pressure Points frequently and the person perks up and feels better fast.

B. The Pressure Points on the face help open up the sinuses. Have tissues nearby as your recipient will drain as you're treating these points!

C. The Pressure Points below the collarbone are over the main "drain" on the chest. When these points are blocked, it "plugs the drain" and keeps congestion in the head, throat and even bronchi. Most recipients report "fluids moving down" after working on these points.

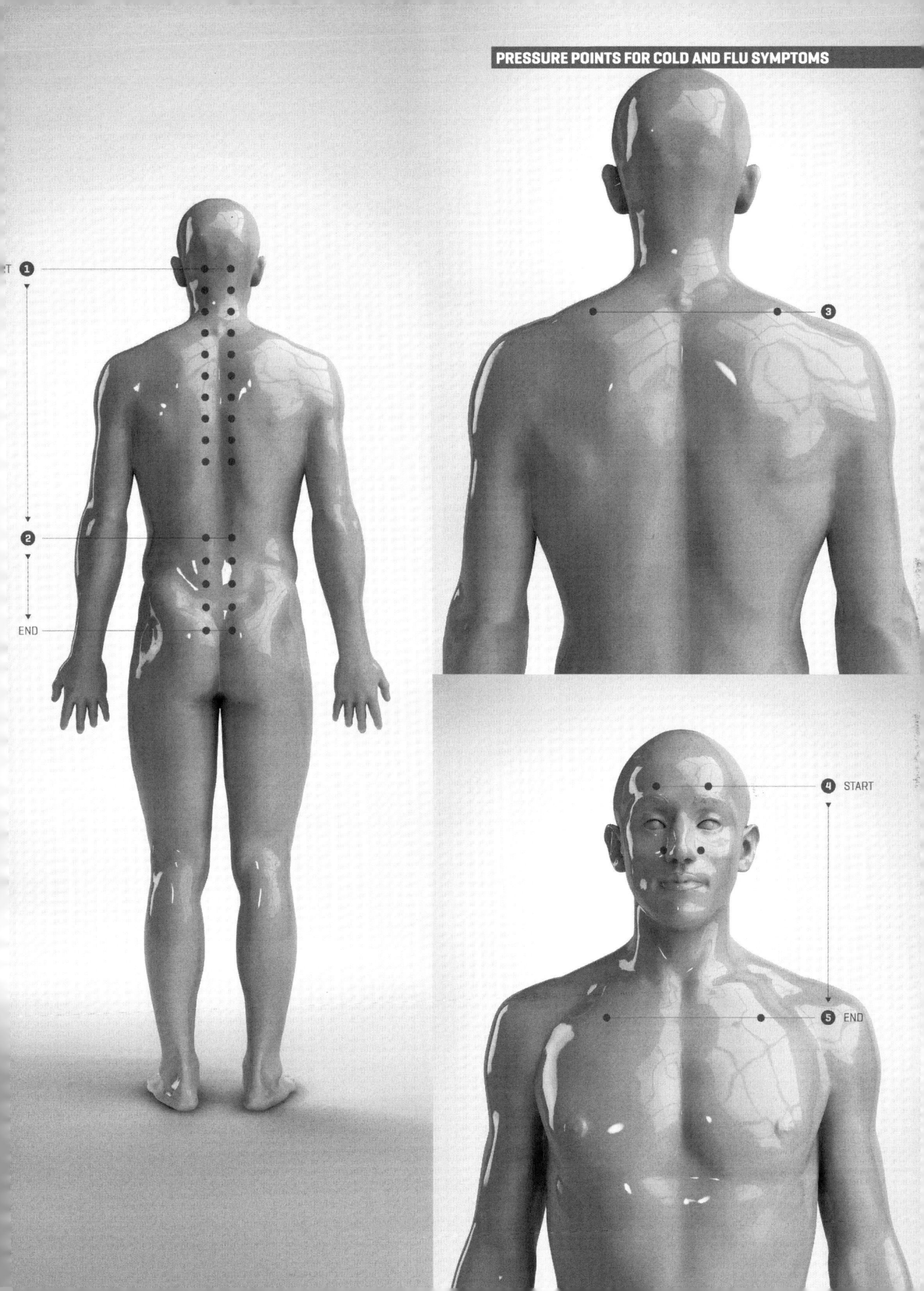

PRESSURE POINTS FOR COLD AND FLU SYMPTOMS

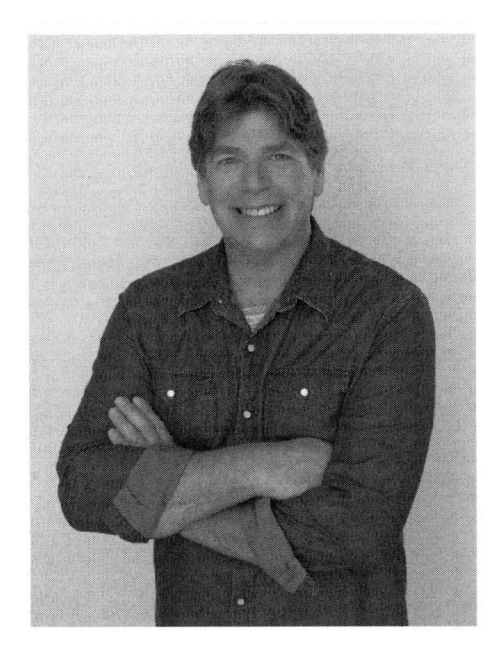

ABOUT THE AUTHOR

Dr. Michael Pinkus was born and raised in Minneapolis, MN. He attended the University of Minnesota and graduated with a Doctor of Chiropractic degree from Northwestern College of Chiropractic in April 1983.

His journey into Alternative Health Care began when he was 17 years old. His initial interest was nutrition, but this branched out into other areas including reflexology and natural health care. In chiropractic college, Dr. Pinkus studied techniques that dated back 4,000 years, including acupuncture, Shiatsu, and other Eastern practices. He also studied Western medicine, with an emphasis on neurology and how the nervous system controls all of the functions of the body.

In 1984, fresh out of college, he began his private practice and quickly expanded it into one of the largest Alternative Health centers in the country. He concurrently began devoting more time to doing public service events, speaking to groups and corporations about health and nutrition. This earned him an honor from the Minnesota Council of Health for his role in Public Health Education.

Seeing the need to expand natural health methods, Dr. Pinkus began touring the country, teaching doctors his techniques. As a result of this, hundreds of doctors are now using Pressure Point Therapy and are getting remarkable results with their patients.

Dr. Pinkus has worked with top Hollywood celebrities and well-known international recording artists. In 1996 he worked as a doctor for the US Men's Wrestling Team in the Atlanta Olympics and has since worked with professional athletes from the NFL, NBA and MLB.

Dr. Pinkus has also been a guest on over 500 radio and TV talk shows across the US, Canada and as far away as South Africa and New Zealand. His own show on Public Television, *Feel Better with Pressure Point Therapy*, began airing in 2016.

"My purpose is to help as many people as I can with Alternative Health Care. As the Latin derivation of the word 'doctor' means teacher, I feel the most important task I can do is to give you useful information that will help yourself, your family and your community."

Yours in Health,

Dr. Michael Pinkus